# color me
# confident

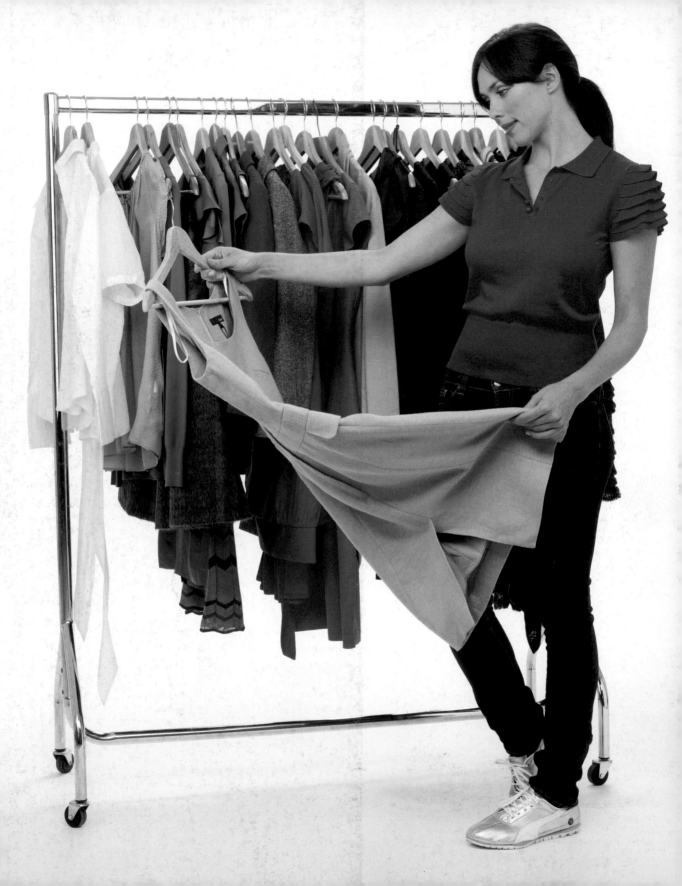

hamlyn

# color me confident

Veronique Henderson
& Pat Henshaw

with 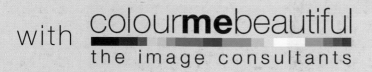 colour**me**beautiful
the image consultants

## DEDICATION

To all **colour me beautiful** consultants for their continued inspiration and support.

An Hachette UK Company
www.hachette.co.uk

First published in Great Britain in 2010 by
Hamlyn, a division of Octopus Publishing Group Ltd
Endeavour House, 189 Shaftesbury Avenue
London WC2H 8JG
www.octopusbooksusa.com

Distributed in the U.S. and Canada by
Octopus Books USA: c/o Hachette Book Group USA,
237 Park Avenue, New York NY 10017

ISBN 978-0-600-61499-9

A CIP catalog recored for this book is available from the Library of Congress.

Printed and bound in China

10 9 8 7 6 5 4 3 2 1

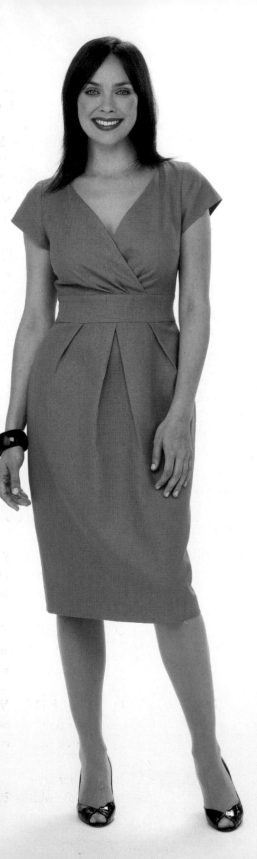

# contents

**INTRODUCTION 6**

1 time for a change 10
Take a fresh look at yourself and discover how to develop a new,
individual style

2 choosing the right colors for you 20
Identify your coloring and find out how to wear a rainbow
of color with confidence

light 34

deep 46

warm 58

cool 70

clear 82

soft 94

3 size doesn't matter, shape does 110
Learn how to emphasize your good points and make
the most of your shape

4 finding your style 144
Express your unique personality through the clothes
you wear and how you wear them

5 pulling it all together 162
Add the finishing touches to your look through hairstyle,
makeup, and accessories

6 making your wardrobe work 192
Reassess your wardrobe and shopping habits to
make sure your clothes suit your lifestyle

**INDEX 204**
**ACKNOWLEDGMENTS 208**

# introduction

OF THE MANY WAYS IN WHICH WE CHOOSE TO EXPRESS OURSELVES, THE COLOR AND STYLE OF OUR CLOTHES PROBABLY MAKE THE MOST IMMEDIATE AND POWERFUL IMPACT. CLOTHES DO NOT SIMPLY COVER THE BODY AND PROTECT US FROM THE ELEMENTS—THEY MAKE A VISUAL STATEMENT ABOUT HOW WE VIEW OURSELVES. CLOTHES REINFORCE OUR SELF-IMAGE AND HELP DEFINE WHO WE ARE. THEY CAN BOOST OUR CONFIDENCE WHEN WE KNOW WE LOOK GOOD, BUT WHEN WE GET IT WRONG, THEY CAN SAP THAT CONFIDENCE JUST AS QUICKLY.

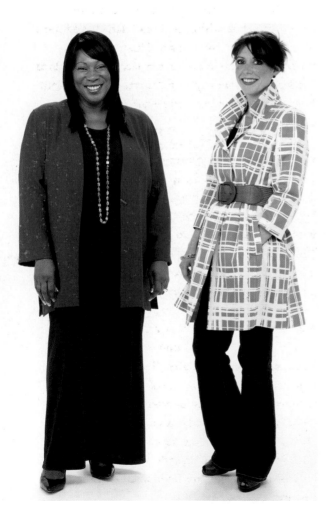

Managing your appearance is an important part of who you are. It tells people about your personality and your lifestyle. Nobody can deny that, in today's world, image matters. We are bombarded with perfect images of actresses and models, and more and more emphasis is placed on looking the part and dressing for success. We all make quick assessments based on how people look. And, while making a judgment on limited information is not the best way to go, it is important to acknowledge that clothing and personal appearance are a form of communication.

Being well dressed does not have to mean dressing expensively or being at the cutting edge of fashion. According to **colour me beautiful**, there are five key points that define a well-dressed woman. Your clothes should:

- Complement your coloring
- Flatter your body lines, scale, and proportions
- Be appropriate
- Match your style personality
- Look current

Whatever your budget, the fashion choices are endless. While increased choice can be exciting, it can be overwhelming and confusing. The key is to know and understand why some pieces work better than others. Forget those fashion faux pas languishing in your closet and look forward to understanding what is special about you.

Clothes are wonderful tools that you can manipulate to present yourself to your advantage, regardless of your size and proportions. By recognizing your physical assets—and limitations—you can explore the many ways in which clothing can be used to draw attention, to conceal, to camouflage, and to create optical illusions. In addition, we are all individuals with a personal style that governs the way we wear our hair, apply makeup, and tie a scarf around our neck.

## all about
## colour me beautiful

For more than 25 years, **colour me beautiful** has been the world's leading image consultancy. Millions of women, including the ubiquitous Bridget Jones, have benefited from "having their colors done." Hot on the heels of *Color Me Confident* (Hamlyn, 2006), we were commissioned to write *Image Matters for Men* (2006), *Color Me Younger* (2008), and *Be a Beautiful Bride* (2009). *Color Me Slimmer* will follow in early 2011. This book is the updated edition of *Color Me Confident*, which tens of thousands of women worldwide have now consulted to learn more about the **colour me beautiful** concepts. The company continues to develop and refine its advice from the original and simple "four seasons" approach to color to a more sophisticated system that encompasses every aspect of your personal image. While color will always be a central theme, it is only one part in developing a personal image and style. You can enjoy taking a fresh look at how to wear colors, rather than simply learning what colors you should wear.

*"The badly dressed woman, people remember the clothes. With a well-dressed woman, they remember the woman."*
Coco Chanel

The consultants at **colour me beautiful**, some of whom are featured in this book, come from all walks of life. Many had other careers before they trained with the organization. They bring with them their collective experiences that make **colour me beautiful** the world's largest and most successful image consultancy. Other women featured in this book have experienced the **colour me beautiful** concept for the first time. They all have one thing in common—they are now confident women.

In addition to working with real women all over the world, **colour me beautiful** has developed programs for clothing stores, since personal shopping is now a popular service offered by many small and large retailers. We also work with corporations on the importance of image in business; we even help members of the automobile industry to sell cars to women. In recent years many consumer goods companies have seen the benefit of adding the services of **colour me beautiful** to their promotional campaigns.

Not a day goes by without a call to our headquarters from the press, TV, or radio requesting information on color, image, and fashion. The questions are varied: Will this new color work for a world-class soccer team? What do you make of this movie star's shoes? So, when it comes to color, style, makeup, and staying current, you are undoubtedly in the best hands possible.

# why buy this book?

The aim of this book is to help you identify the best colors for you to wear and to acknowledge your body lines, scale, and proportions. Armed with this knowledge, along with a sense of your "style personality," you will have the confidence to build a wardrobe that is practical, professional, and/or as glamorous as you need it to be. You will learn that, to meet the demands of your lifestyle, your wardrobe does not have to bulge; it just needs balance. It will become easy for you to shop efficiently, to avoid disaster purchases, and to enjoy yourself more in the whole process.

Basically, you want a wardrobe that works for you. There are many demands on our lives, and having clothes suitable for all occasions can often be beyond our budget and against our inclinations. A coordinated wardrobe takes a little planning, forethought, and a strong will to avoid impulse buys. Following the guidelines in this book will keep you on the straight and narrow without taking the fun out of shopping (for those of you who enjoy it) and without making it a torment (for those who don't).

The right selection of clothes will not only make you look great physically but also help you feel good about yourself—and therefore you become more confident. Wearing the right colors and flattering styles can put a smile on your face, lift your spirits, and improve your outlook.

# how does this book work?

This book is not about changing your physical appearance (though sometimes a little exercise and diet might help). It will not recommend liposuction, Botox, or any kind of surgery. The aim is to bring out the best in you, just as the team of **colour me beautiful** consultants around the world have done every day over the past 25 years for millions of happy, confident women from all walks of life.

Does your lifestyle allow you the time and budget to visit the hairdresser twice a week? Can you spend a fortune on clothes? Do you have endless time to go shopping for clothes while juggling a full-time job, children, a partner, a dog, a garden, and a social life? In this book you will get hints and tips on how to make the most of yourself with minimal effort and budget.

The heart of the book guides you to your dominant color palette—be it light, deep, warm, cool, clear, or soft—then fine-tunes it to the secondary characteristic—warm or cool, soft or clear. Armed with your palette of colors, you are encouraged to assess and learn more about your shape, your proportions, and your "style personality," and to choose and wear your clothes accordingly, and with confidence.

# why **colour me beautiful**?

### IT WILL GIVE YOU CONFIDENCE

- Wearing the right color and style of clothes will make you look younger and healthier.
- Knowing how to adapt your wardrobe for different lifestyles increases your self-esteem (along with making the most of your purchases).
- By adapting your look, staying current, and developing your own individual style, you will feel more confident.

### IT WILL MAKE YOU UNIQUE

No two women will have exactly the same coloring, size and shape, scale and proportions, personality, or budget. But it's useful to have some guidelines to help you make sense of all the choices and focus on what you really need.

Your unique style—the way you wear your hair, your clothes, and how they reflect your lifestyle—is dictated by your personality. With the help of **colour me beautiful**, you stay the same you—but become more confident.

## IT WILL HELP YOU MAKE THE MOST OF YOUR SHAPE

All women wish for the perfect body, but, unfortunately, nature is not always as kind as we would like. With some simple tricks and tips from **colour me beautiful**, any woman can improve her appearance, regardless of her size.

## IT WILL HELP YOU SHOP SUCCESSFULLY

With so many demands on our lives, having suitable clothes for every occasion can often be beyond our reach. With a little forethought and some willpower, you will learn to avoid impulse and unwise buys, and have a closet that works all year round. By following some simple guidelines, the days of a closet full of clothes but nothing to wear will be gone. Learn the secrets that **colour me beautiful** clients discover every day in consultants' studios.

*Once you know you look good, you are ready to face the world—or any situation that calls for poise and control*

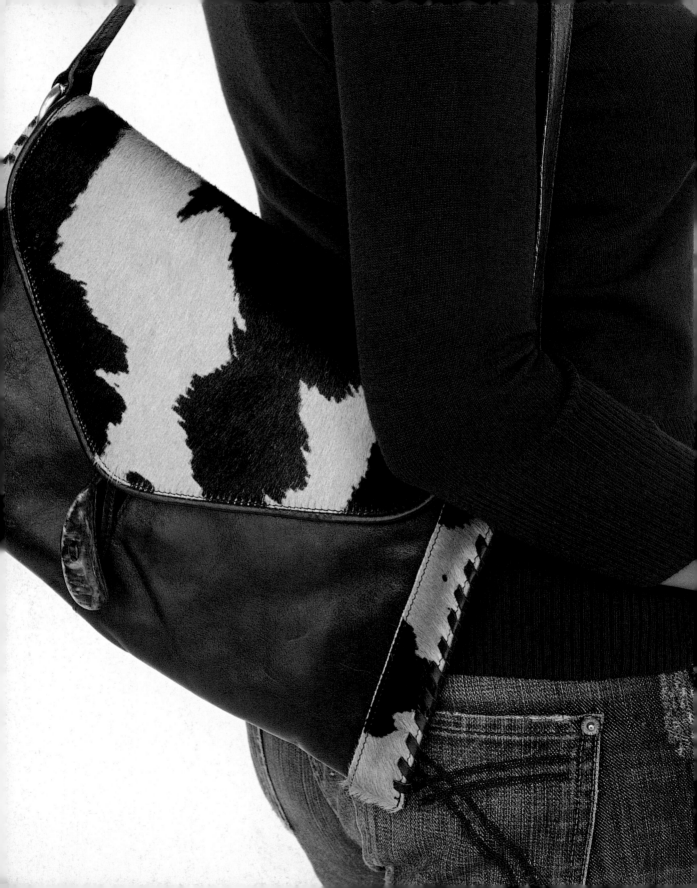

# 1

# time for a change

# take a fresh look

FOR WHATEVER REASON—PERHAPS A NEW JOB, YOUR CHILDREN LEAVING HOME, OR MEETING A NEW PARTNER—
THERE ARE PERIODS IN EVERY WOMAN'S LIFE WHEN THE CLOTHES THAT ALWAYS SEEMED RIGHT JUST DON'T DO
THE JOB ANYMORE. THIS IS THE TIME TO TAKE A FRESH LOOK AT YOURSELF AND TO DEVELOP A STYLE THAT IS
UNIQUELY YOUR OWN.

*Did you know that when you meet someone for the first time you have only 30 seconds to make a lasting impression?*

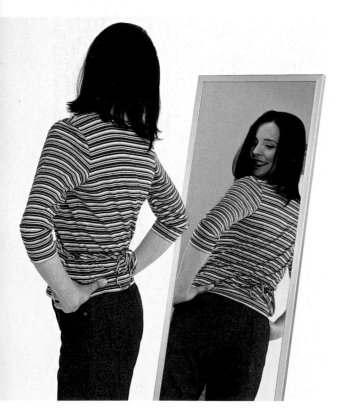

Every day you meet new people, and some of them may become friends—or even enemies. Do you feel confident when you meet someone for the first time? Only 7 percent of a person's judgment of you is based on what you say to them. The rest of their judgment is based on your appearance and body language. So, when you are getting ready to meet new people, do you know exactly what to wear, or do you end up with a pile of clothes on the bedroom floor and wearing your old favorites? Try this confidence test.

## the confidence test
Stand (fully dressed) in front of the mirror, then:
  1 Look at yourself
  2 Smile
  3 Pay yourself a compliment

If you find this easy to do, then congratulations. It is more likely, however, that you will have found only faults: that you're not tall enough/your legs are too short/your hair is lifeless. But how many women who wish for longer legs actually have wonderfully long bodies? Likewise, some women may complain that their waists are too big, even though they invariably have small bottoms and hips. This book will help you start to look at yourself in a new, more positive way.

## START BY FILLING IN THE QUESTIONNAIRE BELOW

**THINGS I LIKE ABOUT MYSELF**

..............................................................................................................
..............................................................................................................
..............................................................................................................
..............................................................................................................
..............................................................................

**THINGS I'D LIKE TO CHANGE**

..............................................................................................................
..............................................................................................................
..............................................................................................................
..............................................................................................................
..............................................................................

**ABOUT COLORS**

◯ Do you wear the same colors every day?

◯ Are there colors that you wear only on weekends?

◯ Are you afraid of color?

◯ Do you tend to wear only black?

**ABOUT SHOPPING**

◯ Do you dislike shopping?

◯ Do you have a closet full of clothes, but nothing to wear?

◯ Do you need a different wardrobe for work?

**ABOUT MAKEUP AND GROOMING**

◯ Have you been applying your makeup in the same way for years?

◯ Have you had the same hairstyle for more than three years?

The items you have checked are the issues on which you need to focus.

For advice on color: **go to pages 20–105**
For help with your closet: **go to pages 192–203**
For makeup and grooming tips: **go to pages 162–183**

# how to use this book

YOU ARE NOT GOING TO CHANGE YOUR LOOK IN AN INSTANT. INSTEAD, YOU WILL FIND THAT YOU WILL USE THIS BOOK AS A MANUAL THAT YOU WILL DIVE INTO OVER A PERIOD OF TIME. ONCE YOU HAVE IDENTIFIED YOUR PRIORITIES FROM THE QUESTIONNAIRE ON THE PREVIOUS PAGE, MAKE ONE OF THEM YOUR STARTING POINT. TAKE IT STEP BY STEP AND BE CONFIDENT WITH EACH STAGE—COLOR, MAKEUP, STYLE, AND ACCESSORIES. OFTEN, **COLOUR ME BEAUTIFUL** CLIENTS WILL ATTEND A COLOR SESSION AND THEN COME BACK A MONTH LATER FOR THE STYLE SESSION. REVISITING A CONCEPT WILL GIVE YOU A FULLER UNDERSTANDING AND THE CONFIDENCE TO GO AHEAD AND USE YOUR NEWFOUND INSIGHT.

There is no miracle solution. While there are some easy tips that will give instant answers, you may need time to take other advice on board. In all cases you have to start with your existing wardrobe—a tweak here and there may be all that is needed—and what your budget allows. Your ultimate aim is to become a confident person who knows how to make the most of herself and who will not hesitate to make a choice when facing her closet every morning.

With sound advice for real women, backed by years of experience from the top **colour me beautiful** team, this book will show you how to achieve the head-to-toe makeover that will give you confidence and change your life. It's up to you now.

## making a change

### STEP 1 – DECISION TIME
- Identify the need for change.
- Prepare yourself for a challenge.

### STEP 2 – COLOR
- Color makes the initial impact, so find out what colors are perfect for you. See Chapter 2, Choosing the Right Colors for You: *go to pages 20–109*.
- By understanding how color is made up, you will see how colors look together and work best to flatter you: *go to pages 22–23*.
- Read about the science of color to understand that although you will have 42 recommended colors, these actually represent thousands of colors that you can wear: *go to pages 24–25*.

### STEP 3 – STYLE
- Take a long look at yourself to establish your basic body shape: *go to pages 112–115*.

- Scale and proportions matter too—and this book shows you why: *go to pages 136–138*.
- From your neck to your ankles, analyze every detail of your body: *go to pages 140–143*.
- Identify your style personality and learn how to enhance it: *go to pages 144–149*.
- Learn which fabrics and textures flatter your body shape—they can make or break an outfit: *go to pages 116–129*.

## STEP 4—SHOPPING HABITS

- Learn how to shop effectively for clothes that look good on you and go together, thus creating a versatile wardrobe: *go to pages 194–203*.
- Whether the thought of shopping leaves you cold or you come to life in the mall, you can learn to use shopping time wisely and to shop efficiently within your budget: *go to pages 196–197*.

## STEP 5—YOUR FACE

- Assess your face shape to make the best choice of hairstyle and glasses: *go to pages 164–170*.
- Follow the makeup application techniques to help you put together a groomed look: *go to pages 171–179*.
- Take notes from the expert advice on makeup, hair, and accessories: *go to pages 164–183*.

## STEP 6—PUTTING IT INTO ACTION

- Pulling it all together: color + body shape + scale + proportions + styling personality + accessories + budget = the real you.

# the well-dressed woman

WHY IS IMAGE SO IMPORTANT? BECAUSE, AS WE HAVE SEEN, IN EVERY WALK OF LIFE WE ARE JUDGED BY OUR APPEARANCE. WHEN YOU FEEL GOOD, YOU ARE MORE CONFIDENT, YOU STAND STRAIGHTER, YOU SMILE MORE, AND YOU EVEN SPEAK WITH MORE CONVICTION.

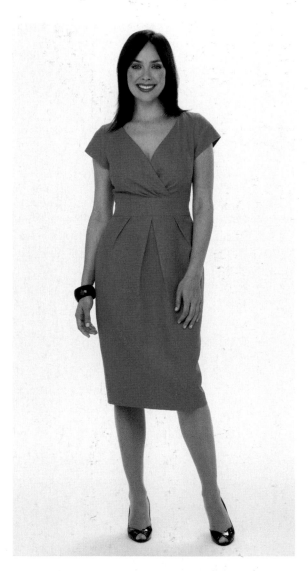

Has anybody ever said to you, "Are you not feeling well today?" when actually you are feeling perfectly fine? It may simply be that you are wearing the wrong color. On the other hand, there may be occasions when you feel tired and stressed but still get complimented. At **colour me beautiful**, we're in the compliment business and we want to make sure that every day you receive compliments about the way YOU look, rather than about the clothes you are wearing.

## the key to success

### COMPLEMENT YOUR COLORING

Your clothes should work in harmony and balance with the coloring of your skin, hair, and eyes. If you are dressed in the right colors, people will see more of you than the clothes you are wearing. Once you understand the right colors and styles for you, you will buy only what suits you when you go shopping. The result will be a more coordinated wardrobe.

### FLATTER YOUR BODY LINES, SCALE, AND PROPORTIONS

You will feel more comfortable wearing clothes that complement your build. An understanding of your basic shape will give you the knowledge to choose clothes that flatter your body line and balance your scale and proportions.

## CHOOSE APPROPRIATE CLOTHES

It is important that your clothes reflect your lifestyle, whether it is professional, casual and relaxed, or formal—or a combination of all three. Not only should your clothes be appropriate for the occasion, you also need to be comfortable in the style of clothes you wear.

## MATCH YOUR STYLE PERSONALITY

You will have a preference for a certain style of clothes, the stores you like to buy from, and the way you accessorize your look. It is your style personality that will pull together the colors, lines, and shape of your clothes.

## LOOK CURRENT

Nothing ages a woman more than clothes that are a decade out of fashion. Fads come and go every year, but trends stay for at least half a decade. The well-dressed woman understands the trends and may use the fads as fun items in her wardrobe.

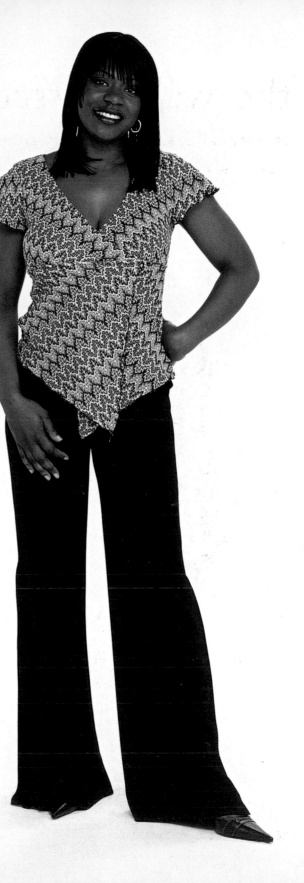

# it could be you

BE INSPIRED BY THESE BEFORE AND AFTER MAKEOVERS. EACH MAKEOVER IS THE RESULT
OF A STEP-BY-STEP PROCESS, AND THROUGH THE NEXT FEW CHAPTERS YOU WILL SEE HOW
THESE WOMEN HAVE TRANSFORMED THEMSELVES.

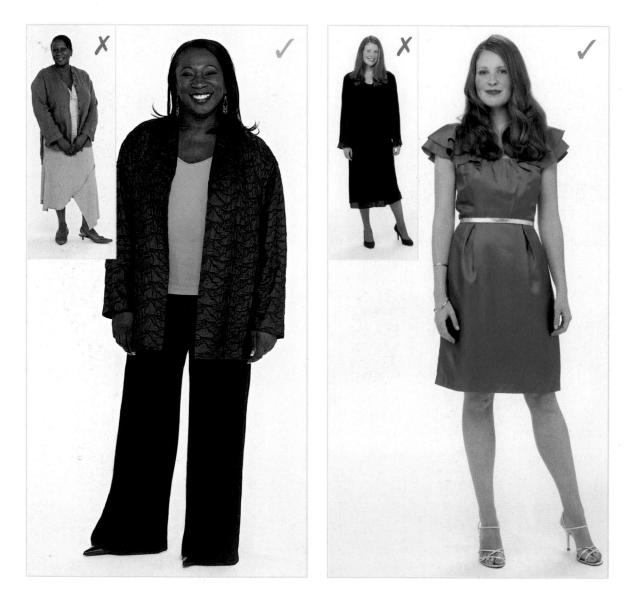

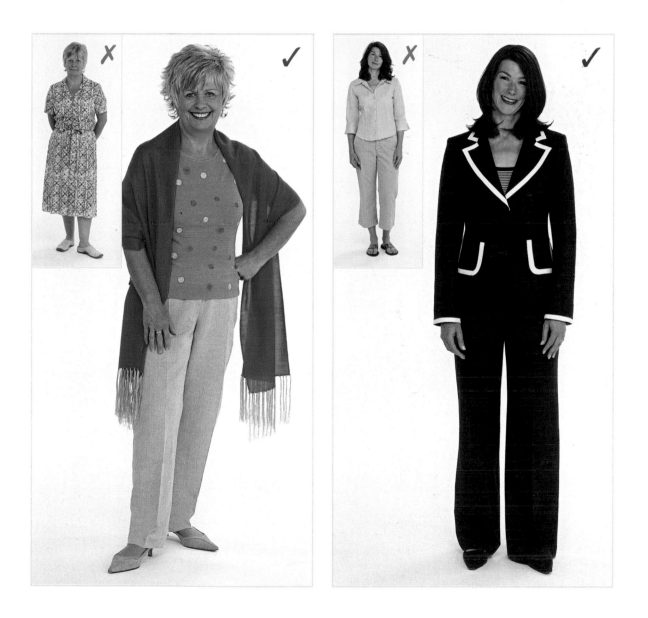

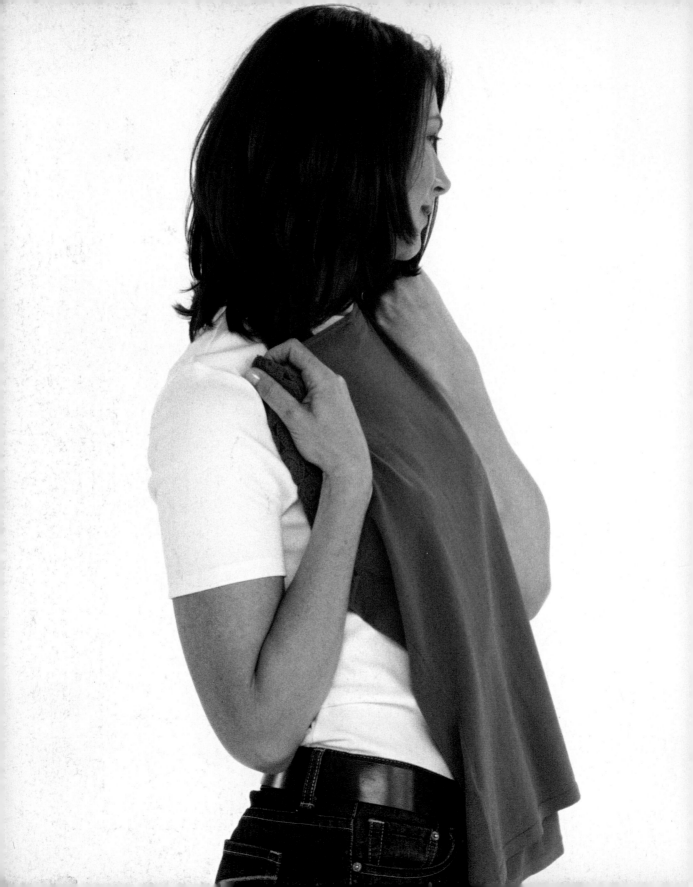

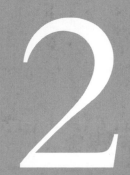

# choosing the right colors for you

# finding your colors

COLOR CAN BE MAGICAL. SEEING A FLASH OF COLOR EMERGE FROM A LARGELY MONOCHROMATIC CROWD IS ENERGIZING, LIKE A BREATH OF FRESH AIR. AND ONCE YOU START WEARING COLORS, THERE WILL BE NO STOPPING YOU. FOR MANY YEARS NEUTRAL COLORS HELD SWAY IN FASHION, BUT NOW THAT COLOR—IN ALL ITS HUES—IS BACK, THE TIME IS RIGHT TO LEARN HOW TO MAKE COLORS WORK FOR YOU. SO LET US TAKE YOU ON A COLORFUL AND STYLISH JOURNEY.

## if you know your coloring

- Shopping will become easier, the choice of colors second nature.
  - You will always have in your wardrobe the right combination of colors to wear.
    - You will gain confidence from knowing that the colors you are wearing are those that flatter.
  - You will be on the exciting path to a new you.

## how color works

When you wear color near your face, the light reflects it upward; this can cast either flattering tones or dark shadows, depending on the mix of the color and your skin tone. This is one reason why it is important to work out your dominant coloring type and discover which are the right colors for you: *go to pages 34–105*.

There is a psychological aspect to color, too, and the colors you wear can communicate nonverbal messages of various kinds. Soft and light tones, for example, will make you appear approachable and friendly, while a red top in the right shade will help give you the confidence you need when facing a stressful situation. Colors that you might wear on a first date with a man you wish to impress will probably not be suitable at a school parents' evening, nor at an important business meeting where you want to appear in control: *go to pages 28–31*.

Once you know what your most flattering colors are, it will be time to concentrate on your choice of accessories and makeup: *go to pages 164–183*. No more guesswork and drawers full of scarves and makeup that you do not wear, without knowing exactly why.

*Most women wear only 20 percent of their wardrobe 80 percent of the time*

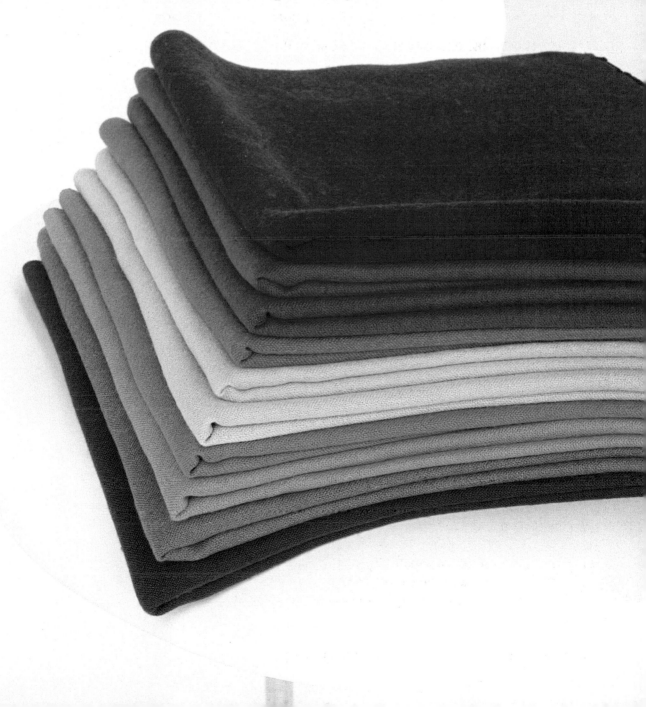

# the science of color

THERE ARE TWO MAIN INFLUENCES BEHIND **COLOR ME BEAUTIFUL'S** CURRENT APPROACH TO COLOR—THOSE OF JOHANNES ITTEN AND ALFRED MUNSELL. THE SEASONAL COLOR CONCEPT THAT LAY BEHIND THE ORIGINAL COLOR ME BEAUTIFUL—AND WHICH LASTED FOR OVER 20 YEARS—WAS FIRST DEVELOPED IN THE 1920S BY THE ARTIST JOHANNES ITTEN OF THE BAUHAUS SCHOOL. ITTEN NOTICED THAT HIS STUDENTS ALWAYS DID THEIR BEST WORK USING COLORS THEY HAD CHOSEN THEMSELVES. IN HIS BOOK *THE ART OF COLOR*, ITTEN REVEALS THE STRONG RELATIONSHIP BETWEEN A STUDENT'S APPEARANCE, THEIR PERSONALITY, AND THE COLORS THEY LIKED TO WORK WITH.

This concept was further developed at the Fashion Academy of Los Angeles, founded in 1972. Former student Carole Jackson made the seasonal concept popular in her book *Color Me Beautiful*, published in 1980. The book was translated into many languages and for months remained on the *New York Times* best-seller list. In 1986 Doris Pooser developed Carole Jackson's seasonal concept further, but with the addition of the Munsell theory (see opposite), in her book *Always in Style*.

The Munsell system was partly responsible for **colour me beautiful** moving from four to twelve seasonal palettes in 1991 with the publication of Mary Spillane's *The Complete Style Guide*. Its inclusion in today's **colour me beautiful** approach gives a more flexible way of using color. The beauty of Munsell's system is that it can be used to describe a person's coloring as well as to specify the colors they should wear, the aim always being to create harmony and balance between the two. The theory behind his system is that all colors have one dominant characteristic and one or two secondary characteristics. A person's coloring will also have one dominant characteristic and, for the purposes of this book, one secondary characteristic. Working with this formula will give women a reliable, versatile, and easy-to-follow way of using color.

# the Munsell system

Munsell's is the most widely accepted system of color measurement; it is used by both the US National Bureau of Standards and the British Standards Institution. So, who was Munsell? In 1903 Albert Munsell—also an artist—invented a system of color identification based on the responses of the human eye. In 1905 his System of Color Notation became universally recognized as the language of color. In this, colors were identified as having three characteristics: hue, value, and chroma.

The uses of this "language" are innumerable, particularly in the building, printing, and automobile industries. The Munsell system is even used to codify all tints and dyes within the hairdressing industry. So if you color your hair, you are already using the Munsell system.

All three Munsell characteristics—**hue**, **value**, and **chroma**—can be referred to when describing a color.

### HUE – UNDERTONE

Hue defines a color's undertone, which may be warm (yellow-based) or cool (blue-based). Colors such as red, pink, and green can be described as having either a warm or a cool undertone. You might have a cool "blue" red (say, a plum-colored red) or a warm "orange" red (a tomato red); likewise, you can have a warm olive green (yellow-based) or a cool pine green (blue-based).

### VALUE – DEPTH

The value of a color refers to its depth, giving a measure of its lightness or darkness. Munsell used a scale of 0 to 10, with black being 0 and white being 10, with all the shades of gray in between. This grading of light and dark can be used to measure the depth of all other colors, too; for example, in hairdressing these numbers determine the depth of color of a hair dye.

### CHROMA – CLARITY

Chroma indicates the purity or clarity of a color. Some colors are bright and vibrant and reflect the light, while others are dusty or muted and seem to absorb light. The type of fabric will also determine whether light is absorbed or reflected; for example, satin reflects light, while wool seems to absorb it. The chroma scale ranges from 0 to 14, with 0 being the most grayed or muted and 14 being the clearest.

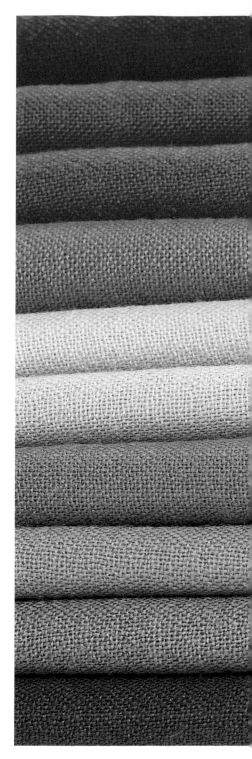

# how does color analysis work?

THE PROCESS OF ANALYSIS LOOKS AT THE UNDERTONE (HUE), DEPTH (VALUE), AND CLARITY (CHROMA) OF DIFFERENT COLORS AGAINST YOUR SKIN, EYES, AND HAIR TO DETERMINE YOUR DOMINANT TYPE. WORK THROUGH THIS SECTION TO DISCOVER YOUR OWN COLORING TYPE.

Color analysis was made popular by **colour me beautiful**. Millions of women have had a color analysis with a fully trained consultant in either a studio or the workplace. When you visit a **colour me beautiful** consultant, they will look at your combination of hair color, eye color, and skin tone. This is the beginning of a process to determine which one of the six dominant coloring types you are—**Light** or **Deep**, **Warm** or **Cool**, **Clear** or **Soft**: *go to pages 34–105*.

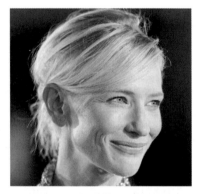

LIGHT

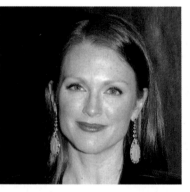

WARM

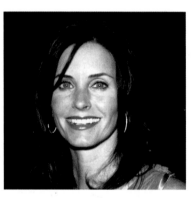

CLEAR

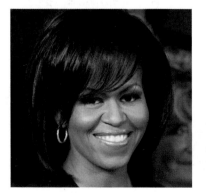

DEEP

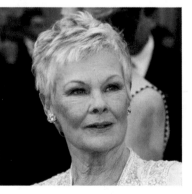

COOL

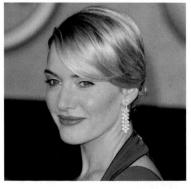

SOFT

# the time of your life

We are all born with perfect skin, beautiful eyes, and healthy hair, the colors of which are all genetically balanced together. Over the years environment, diet, and everyday stresses can all take their toll on how we look. You may, for example, live in a climate where your natural hair color becomes sun-streaked and your skin acquires an olive tone.

When the hormones start up—first in your teens and then again at the time of menopause—it all changes again. If you look at a photograph of yourself as a young child, and then as a teenager, you may well see a marked difference in hair color. The gorgeous platinum blonde child has now become a young woman with dark blonde hair.

That young woman matures gracefully into an ash-gray grandmother. In addition, of course, she may have played with nature during countless trips to a colorist at the hairdressers. Similarly, a beautiful red mane will gently fade and possibly even go gray, while the head of striking ebony hair will be the one to show early signs of white. Skin tone will have been affected by those hormones, as well as by climate, diet, and lifestyle. As we age, our eye color may also lighten and soften.

If you were color analyzed some years ago, you may now have changed and feel less happy wearing certain recommended colors. For this reason, the idea that a person is one "season" or palette all their life is no longer true.

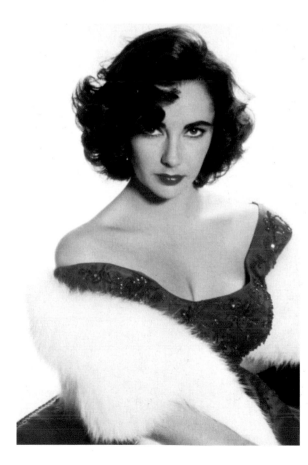

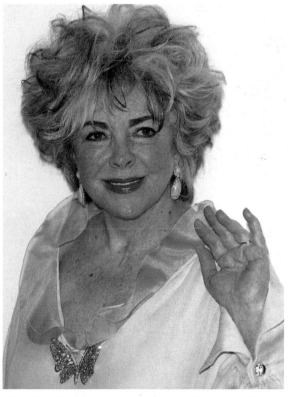

*Elizabeth Taylor's coloring went from Clear and Warm in her youth to Soft and Cool as she reached her sixties.*

# the psychology of color

MUCH RESEARCH HAS BEEN DONE ON THE PSYCHOLOGY OF COLOR AND ITS EFFECTS ON EVERYDAY LIFE. COLOR CAN AFFECT YOUR MOOD AND YOUR ENERGY LEVELS PROFOUNDLY, AND THEREFORE HAS A GREAT IMPACT ON YOUR GENERAL SENSE OF WELL-BEING. IT WILL ALSO AFFECT HOW OTHERS VIEW YOU, FROM YOUR PARTNER TO YOUR BOSS.

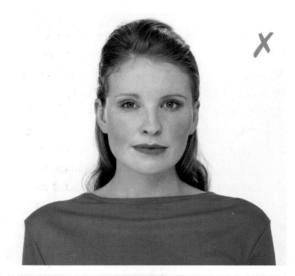

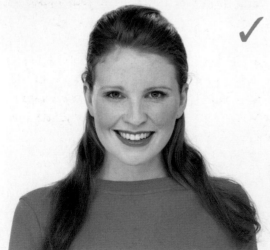

Before you get to find out about your own coloring type, let us first take a look at the psychological effect on yourself and others when you wear certain colors: *go to pages 29–31*. This is not gleaned from the results of scientific research but from the knowledge and vast experience that **colour me beautiful** has gained over the years in the course of meeting so many women.

## investment buys

For each of the six dominant coloring types, we have suggested—and commented on—the best colors for investment buys. These are the items that you want to remain in your wardrobe for as long as possible, as opposed to the fun tops and sandals that you are happy to wear for just a few months. Investment buys are most likely to be coats, jackets, and slacks; they could also be a fabulous cashmere sweater or even a handbag.

*The blue undertone of the hot pink top casts dark shadows onto her face, while the yellow-based terracotta top lights up her complexion, giving her a healthy glow.*

## BLACK/GRAY

*Black can portray an air of authority, and it is worn by many women as a uniform for business*

Wearing black from head to toe every day is easy and safe, but may give the message that you lack imagination. It also implies that you are hiding behind the color. It might be a good idea to wear black with another color for greater impact. For example, a little black evening dress can be a winner; if black is not in your palette, wear it with accessories near your face (pearls or beads) that tone well with your natural coloring. A pashmina or chiffon scarf in your colors will be perfect. Or, you could wear a suitable gray—either charcoal, medium gray, or pewter—instead.

## BROWN

*Brown, the color of the earth, is a great color to wear when you're in a relaxed mode*

The brown family comes in many guises: chocolate, coffee, mahogany, and golden, to name just a few. Brown denotes a friendly, down-to-earth, though serious, attitude. We are often told that brown is "this season's black," and it provides an excellent alternative for those with Warm coloring, especially when you want to appear less threatening. Brown may be considered boring when worn on its own, but mixing it with other colors can bring it to life, and it could become a staple of your casual and work wardrobe.

Make sure you choose the correct shade for you by checking which tone of brown is in your dominant palette.

## BEIGE

*This family of colors is a great substitute for black and browns in the summer*

The beiges run from stone to camel via taupe, pewter, cocoa, and natural. All of these tones are nonthreatening, friendly, and approachable; they are excellent when you want people to open up to you. They are ideal colors for anyone who works with people, for example in counseling, human resources, or nursing.

If your coloring is either Deep (pages 46–57) or Clear (pages 82–93), beige generally needs to be worn together with contrasting colors.

The joy of these tones is that they can be worn all year round with the fashion colors from your palette.

## WHITE

*White denotes purity and freshness*

Everyone needs white in their palette, whether worn head to toe for a special outing or as a contrast against other colors from your palette. It can be a hard color to wear in its purest form, but there are shades of white to suit everyone, from soft white to ivory and cream; once you have identified your dominant coloring type on the following pages, refer to your color palette to see which shade is best for you.

Wearing white in a textured fabric will often soften its appearance. Linen and silk, for example, are rarely a pure white, although cotton can be. White is an ideal color to wear in hot climates, because it reflects light—the challenge is keeping it clean and fresh-looking.

## BLUE

*Blue, the color of logic, activates the mind*

Blue conveys trust, peace, and order—it could be considered safe. When a leading British scarf retailer commissioned a survey to find out which colors sold best, blue came out on top. Dark navy is often associated with authority and law and order; many police forces use navy for their uniforms.

Medium shades of blue, such as cornflower, lapis, and sapphire, are all great colors to brighten up your wardrobe throughout the year. The lighter shades, such as powder blue, eau de nil, bluebell, and sky blue, make wonderful colors for special occasions when a feminine look may be required. Teamed with darker shades (navy and gray), they become great colors for shirts and tops.

## PINK

*Wearing pink suggests gentleness and empathy; it brings out the femininity in every woman*

All women need some pink in their wardrobe, whether it is for a robe, some underwear, or a pashmina. Wearing a powder pink outfit will not be your most powerful look, but a blush pink or cyclamen pink worn under a business suit will give you authority. Or, wow them on the dance floor with any shade of pink from apricot to fuchsia— but not worn head to toe.

Pink is a great color to wear when you are feeling a little off-color, because it gives a flattering lift to any complexion.

## PURPLE

*In its pure form, purple shows creativity as well as indicating sensitivity*

The purple family runs from softest lavender to deepest damson. It is a great alternative—and a more exciting one—to black and navy. But be careful that its creative signal does not compromise a situation where you want to appear to conform. Purple is also the color of spirituality and meditation. In its lighter forms, the lilacs and soft violets promote a general sense of relaxation.

Many people steer clear of purple, but if you've never worn it, give it a try in a scarf or pashmina. You'll be amazed at the effect it has on others.

## RED

*Red is the color of energy; wear red and you will feel confident and in control*

The red family has many variations, from raspberry to tomato, so getting the undertone right is crucial. Is it warm (yellow-based) or cool (blue-based)?

Wearing red will bring excitement into your day. It is the color of stimulation, showing a sense of exhilaration but also suggesting a demanding character. It is a great color to wear at the end of the week, when your energy levels may be flagging. Do not, however, wear red when trying to calm children at bedtime.

When wearing red, take care with choosing your lipstick. Make sure it is in the same tone, although it can be lighter or darker.

## GREEN

*Green, the color of grass and leaves, conveys a sense of calm and reassurance*

When wearing green, whether olive or lime, or anything in between, you show creativity and imagination. It was once thought to be unlucky, but in the world of fashion, green brings another dimension to the wardrobe. With all its various shades, green may be used for virtually any garment, from a winter coat to a fun pair of shoes.

With green, it is particularly important to understand the undertone and to know whether you are better in a warm (yellow-based) green, such as moss or apple green, or the cool (blue-based) green of spruce or sea green.

# gaining color confidence

ALL YOU NEED TO DO TO DETERMINE WHICH ARE THE BEST COLORS FOR YOU IS TO FOLLOW THE SIMPLE STEPS
OUTLINED BELOW. THESE ARE COVERED IN MORE DETAIL IN THE FOLLOWING SECTIONS ON EACH COLORING TYPE:
LIGHT, DEEP, WARM, COOL, CLEAR, AND SOFT.

### STEP 1 – FINDING YOUR DOMINANT COLORING

Look through the following pages and decide
which of our celebrities' coloring most closely
resembles yours.

- Do you have light hair and light eyes?
  *Go to page 34*.
- Do you have dark hair and dark eyes?
  *Go to page 46*.
- Does your hair have red tones?
  *Go to page 58*.
- Do you have gray tones in your hair?
  *Go to page 70*.
- Is your hair dark, but your eyes light?
  *Go to page 82*.
- Or are you a mixture of all?
  *Go to page 94*.

Once you have identified the celebrity, you
will know your dominant coloring type. Read
through that section (Light, Deep, Warm and so
on) to understand how your 30 best colors will
work for you.

### STEP 2 – FINDING YOUR SECONDARY CHARACTERISTIC

Now see if there is a definite undertone of warm
or cool to your skin. Look at the underside of
your arm (which will not be sun-damaged). Warm
skins have a yellow undertone, while cool skins are
pinkish. The best way to see this is by doing a
comparison test with your friends. Some people
will show neither a warm nor cool undertone to
their skin—they have a neutral skin. If you have a
natural tan, this should not affect the undertone.

*A dominant Light coloring is
indicated by blonde hair and pale
eyes and skin; golden tones to hair
and skin indicate a secondary
characteristic of Warm.*

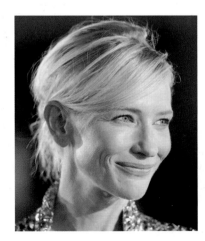 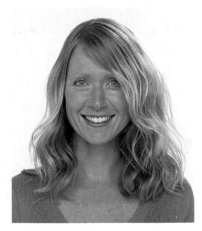

# the color test

Within the sections for each dominant coloring type—Light, Deep, Warm, Cool, Clear, and Soft—there are two subsections. Each subsection suggests different colors to try against your skin in order to determine your secondary color characteristic: *go to pages 34–105*.

Find examples of the suggested colors, using scarves, tops, or any other garment that you can easily hold near your face. If necessary, borrow from your friends—you could also ask for their help in deciding which of the colors under scrutiny are best for you.

Sit in front of a mirror with no makeup on. Make sure you are in a well-lit area, with no shadows falling on your face. Natural daylight is preferable. Hold each of the suggested colors in turn under your chin and look at the result. Does the color show on your chin? Does the color make your complexion change?

## YOU'LL KNOW THE COLOR IS RIGHT WHEN:

- Your face appears to be lit from underneath.
- Your skin appears smoother, fresher, and younger; lines and blemishes are minimized.
- Your eye color is enhanced.
- You notice YOU more than the color.

## YOU'LL IDENTIFY THE WRONG COLORS WHEN:

- There are dark or colored shadows around your chin and neck.
- Your complexion looks uneven in color.
- The color stands out more than you.

You can now focus on your secondary characteristic, which adds 12 additional colors to your 30 dominant colors, giving 42 colors that you can use with confidence, in the knowledge that these are the right choices for you.

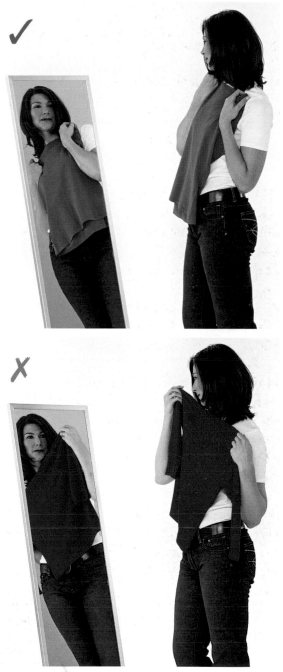

*For someone who is a Deep and Warm, the color test will reveal that salmon is a more flattering shade of pink than fuchsia.*

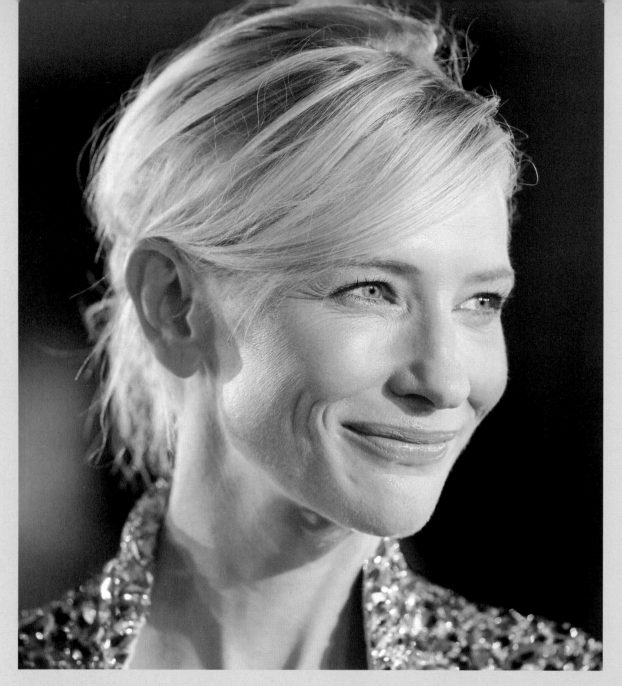

# light

With her pale blonde hair, porcelain skin, and blue eyes, Australian actress Cate Blanchett is an archetypal Light.

# are you a light?

## do you have...
- Naturally blonde or very light hair?
- Pale blue, gray, or light green eyes?
- Pale eyelashes?
- Pale or indistinguishable eyebrows that you often pencil in?
- Delicate skin, probably porcelain in tone, that burns easily in the sun?

## your look is
- Light and delicate.
- The undertone of your skin may be either warm or cool.
- The depth of your coloring is light.
- The clarity of your look may be either clear or soft.

## your ideal colors
For a master color palette: *go to pages 36–37*.

## how to wear your colors
Balance your dominant look by wearing light or medium-depth color near your face. If you have to choose a darker tone, such as light navy, for a jacket, try to contrast it with a light shade such as light apricot, rather than with a deep one like geranium.

Wear two light colors together or a combination of light and dark—but never wear two dark colors together. Always aim to have the lighter colors close to your face.

## be careful
Shopping may be a challenge in the winter season, especially when you are looking for a coat or jacket, since these are traditionally dark in color. Try rose brown—or wear a scarf or pashmina in a light shade over your coat.

## investment buys
When it comes to buying items that you expect to keep for more than a season or two, the colors below are great substitutes for black. They do not date, and you can wear them all year.

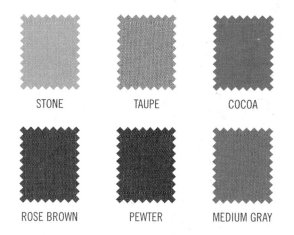

STONE  TAUPE  COCOA

ROSE BROWN  PEWTER  MEDIUM GRAY

Now find out whether you are
Light and Warm: **go to page 38** or
Light and Cool: **go to page 42**.

# light color palette

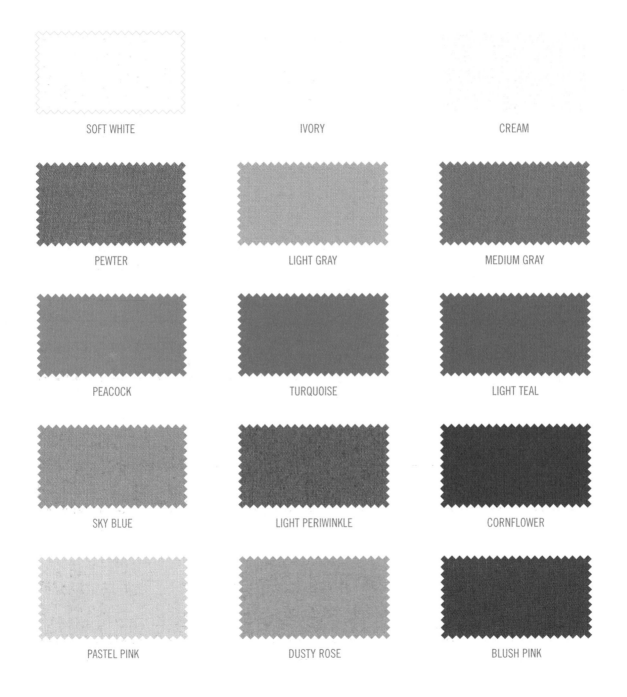

SOFT WHITE

IVORY

CREAM

PEWTER

LIGHT GRAY

MEDIUM GRAY

PEACOCK

TURQUOISE

LIGHT TEAL

SKY BLUE

LIGHT PERIWINKLE

CORNFLOWER

PASTEL PINK

DUSTY ROSE

BLUSH PINK

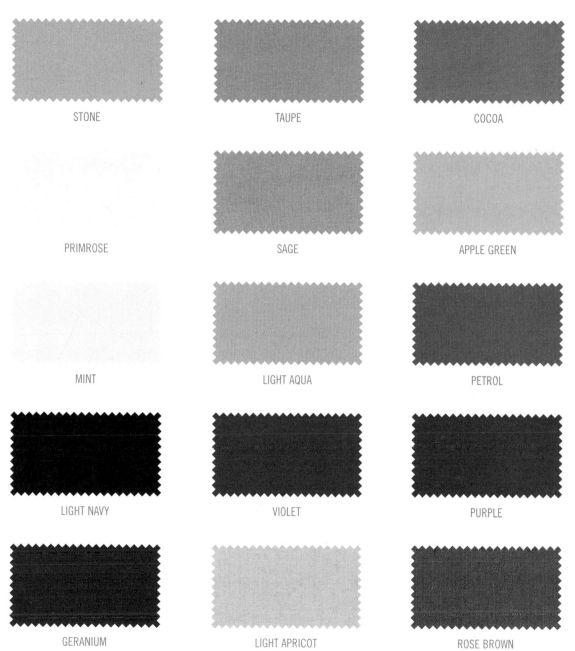

STONE

TAUPE

COCOA

PRIMROSE

SAGE

APPLE GREEN

MINT

LIGHT AQUA

PETROL

LIGHT NAVY

VIOLET

PURPLE

GERANIUM

LIGHT APRICOT

ROSE BROWN

# light & warm

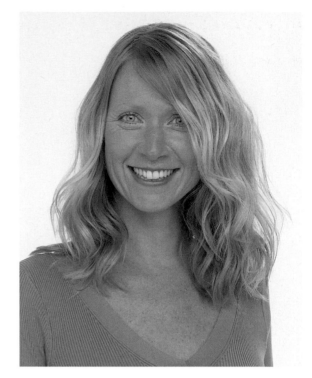

- Take a close look at your hair color. When you are in sunlight or under a spotlight, do you see warm or strawberry-blonde tints in your hair?
- Does your skin have a golden tone?
- Do your eyes have a brightness to them?
- Do the color test with peach and powder pink, and with light moss and sea green: *go to page 33*. You should find that your best pink is peach, a warm shade with yellow undertones, while the light moss will suit you better than the sea green.

Your secondary characteristic is warm. There is a clarity to your additional colors that will complement your bright eyes.

## your additional colors

As a Light and Warm, you can now add these 12 extra shades to your master palette. Notice that they all have a warm (yellow) undertone; avoid wearing icy shades and colors with a strong blue undertone. The grays and navy in your master palette are best worn with peach, yellow-green, and lemon.

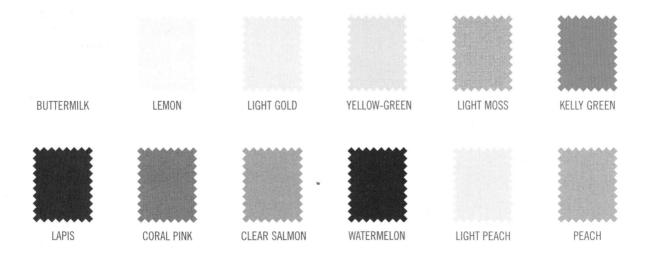

| BUTTERMILK | LEMON | LIGHT GOLD | YELLOW-GREEN | LIGHT MOSS | KELLY GREEN |
| LAPIS | CORAL PINK | CLEAR SALMON | WATERMELON | LIGHT PEACH | PEACH |

# in your makeup bag

**EYE PENCIL**   COFFEE

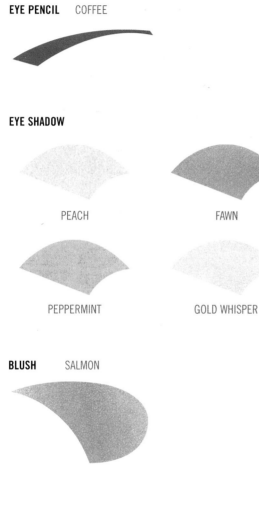

**EYE SHADOW**

PEACH

FAWN

PEPPERMINT

GOLD WHISPER

**BLUSH**   SALMON

**LIP PENCIL**   NATURAL

**LIPSTICK**   WARM PINK

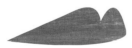

CORAL

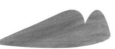

WARM SAND

# your face

- The overall look of your makeup should be light and subtle. Do not overpower your delicate, warm complexion with dark, strong shades for eye shadow or lipstick.
- For eye pencils try coffee; you might also like teal or moss green.
- Accent eye shadows in light shades of green and orange such as peppermint and fawn will work well when blended with gold whisper or peach.
- Keep your blush warm-toned, using a color such as salmon.
- Lip pencils should be kept light and pale; natural is a good choice, since it will not deepen your lipstick color.
- Finish your look with lipstick colors such as warm pink, warm sand, coral, or peachy tones, and avoid dark, muted browns.

# your hair

- Of all the dominant colorings, your naturally blonde hair will need the least help through the addition of color, though you may wish to add a few golden tones to enhance the texture; avoid the temptation to go dark.
- When the natural highlights that come with age start to show, go for an all-over color that will give the appearance of golden highlights.

# mixing colors with confidence light & warm

## warm-weather combinations

## cool-weather combinations

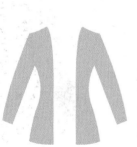

### BUSINESS WEAR
sage + light peach
light gray + light gold
taupe + yellow-green
cornflower +
clear salmon

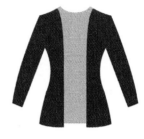

### BUSINESS WEAR
light navy + peach
rose brown + buttermilk
pewter + light moss
medium gray +
coral pink

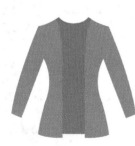

### CASUAL WEAR
apple green + buttermilk
light aqua + mint
light moss + pastel pink
blush pink +
light periwinkle

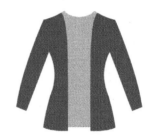

### CASUAL WEAR
petrol + peach
watermelon + cream
light teal + lapis
cornflower +
yellow-green

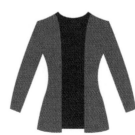

### SPECIAL OCCASION WEAR
turquoise + light teal
light periwinkle + lapis
coral pink + peach
kelly green +
yellow-green

### SPECIAL OCCASION WEAR
lapis + sky blue
violet + purple
geranium + coral pink
kelly green +
yellow-green

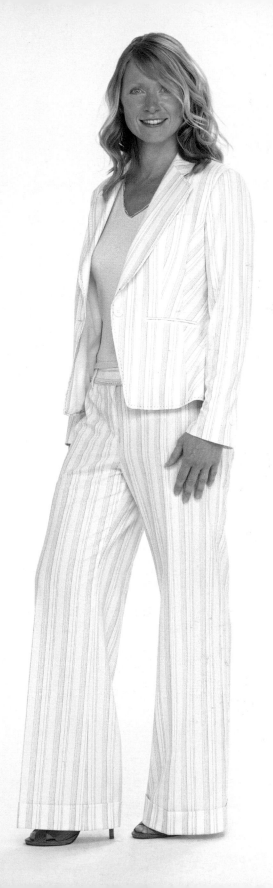

**LEFT** *The perfect combination for someone who is Light and Warm is two light shades worn together.*

## ALTERNATIVE TO BLACK

The key to getting your look right as a Light and Warm is to make sure that you always wear light shades near your face. So for a flattering look for work, rose brown, cocoa, and pewter make the prefect substitute for black or very dark colors. Of course, your light navy, petrol, and purple are also great colors, but remember to wear them with something light. Don't forget to avoid wearing two dark colors together.

Now that you know your color palette, find out how to reflect your style through color: **go to pages 144–161**.

# light & cool

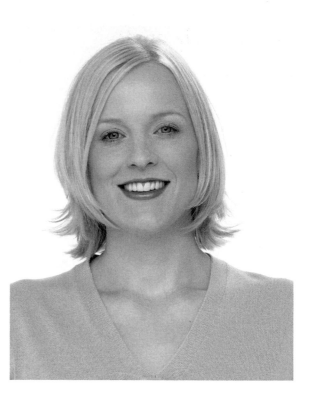

- Take a close look at your hair color under good light. Does it have light ash tints?
- Does your skin have a pinkish tone?
- Do your eyes have a pale, misty appearance?
- Do the color test with peach and powder pink, and with light moss and sea green: *go to page 33*. You should find that your best pink is powder pink, which has a cool undertone, while the sea green will suit you better than the light moss.

Your secondary characteristic is cool. Notice that there is a muted appearance to your additional colors, which will complement your eyes.

## your additional colors

As a Light and Cool, you can add these 12 extra shades to your master palette; all have a cool (blue) undertone. Avoid warm shades and colors with a strong yellow undertone. Primrose or apple green from your master palette will look stunning with gray or navy.

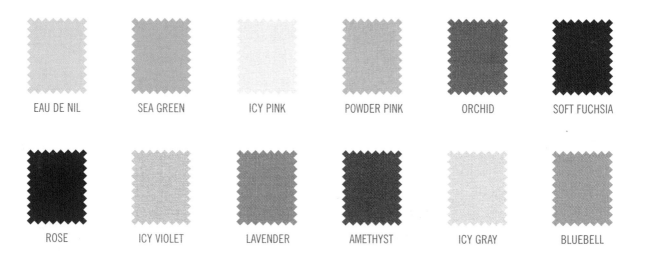

| EAU DE NIL | SEA GREEN | ICY PINK | POWDER PINK | ORCHID | SOFT FUCHSIA |
| --- | --- | --- | --- | --- | --- |
| ROSE | ICY VIOLET | LAVENDER | AMETHYST | ICY GRAY | BLUEBELL |

# in your makeup bag

**EYE PENCIL**   GRANITE

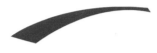

**EYE SHADOW**

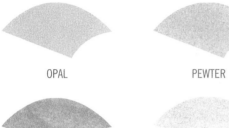

OPAL                    PEWTER

LILAC                    PEARL

**BLUSH**   ROSE

**LIP PENCIL**   NATURAL

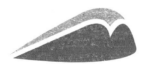

**LIPSTICK**   DUSTY ROSE

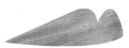

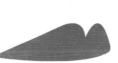

PINK SHELL              BONBON

# your face

- The overall look of your makeup should be light and subtle. Do not overpower your delicate complexion with strong, dark shades for eye shadow or lipstick.
- For eye pencils try granite, amethyst, or dark blue.
- Accent eye shadows like pewter, lilac, or pearl will blend well with opal or pale pink.
- Keep your blush pale, but make it a cool color such as rose or candy pink.
- Lip pencils should be kept light: try natural.
- Since your coloring is light and cool, the best lipsticks will be pale soft pinks and light mauves such as dusty rose, pink shell, and bonbon; avoid coral or salmon shades.

# your hair

- Your hair is naturally ash blonde, so any color that you add to it will need to be either ash or platinum.
- When gray highlights start to appear as you age, they will lift the existing base tone of your hair and you will go gray beautifully—so you may prefer not to add any color to it and let nature take its course.
- Avoid the temptation to add warm tones to your hair.

# mixing colors with confidence light & cool

## warm-weather combinations

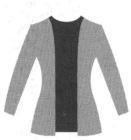

**BUSINESS WEAR**
light gray + icy violet
taupe + orchid
bluebell + eau de nil
cocoa + powder pink

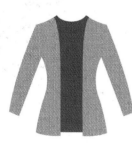

**CASUAL WEAR**
sky blue + rose
geranium + icy gray
peacock + sea green
blush pink + icy pink

**SPECIAL OCCASION WEAR**
lavender + violet
sea green + mint
light aqua + eau de nil
powder pink + orchid

## cool-weather combinations

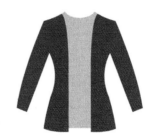

**BUSINESS WEAR**
light navy + bluebell
petrol + sea green
pewter + icy pink
medium gray + orchid

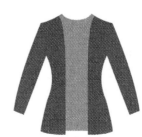

**CASUAL WEAR**
purple + powder pink
amethyst + pastel pink
light teal + light aqua
light periwinkle +
lavender

**SPECIAL OCCASION WEAR**
amethyst + lavender
geranium + icy gray
turquoise + sea green
bluebell +
light periwinkle

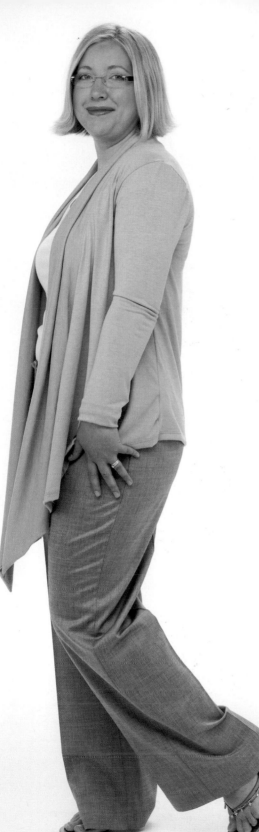

**LEFT** *A combination of light and cool tones works best on someone who is Light and Cool.*

## ALTERNATIVE TO BLACK

Your delicate Light and Cool coloring means you have to think carefully about the types of colors you use as an alternative to black. Staying with the light neutrals in your palette is the answer. Medium gray, sky blue, and amethyst make a perfect combination for you. If your work look is very formal, then light navy, pewter, and even purple are good alternatives.

Now that you know your color palette, find out how to reflect your style through color: **go to pages 144–161**.

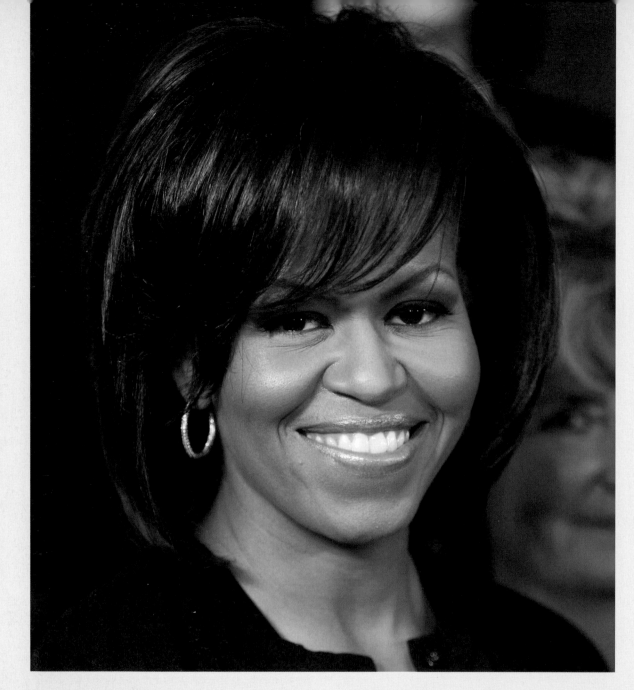

# deep

*With her dark eyes and hair, Michelle Obama represents the true coloring of Deep women.*

# are you a deep?

## do you have...
- Dark brown to black hair?
- Dark eyes?
- Dark eyebrows and lashes?
- Skin tone from porcelain to black, including all the shades in between?

## your look is
- Dark and strong.
- The undertone of your skin may be either warm or cool.
- Your overall look is deep.
- You may be clear or soft.

## your ideal colors
For a master color palette: *go to pages 48–49*.

## how to wear your colors
You can wear black on its own, or team it with dark shades such as black-brown and eggplant for day or royal purple for a sophisticated look. If you are a Dramatic type (pages 152–153), try black with a single bold color such as scarlet.

To balance your look, wear strong, dark colors near your face. Contrast these with lighter or brighter shades from your palette. Wear two dark colors, or light and dark, but never choose two light colors.

## be careful
In a warmer climate you may be tempted to go for lighter shades, but be careful when wearing pale or pastel shades on their own. These will always look better on you when worn with dark

or bright colors for contrast. Be bold and choose brighter colors from your palette such as lime, emerald green, turquoise, or blush pink, and combine them with stone or taupe. Remember to wear the stronger colors near your face. If you decide to wear light shades near your face, balance your look with deeper-colored makeup so that you don't look pale and washed out.

## investment buys
For the items that will have longevity in your wardrobe, choose the colors below and wear them with a darker or brighter contrast:

BLACK

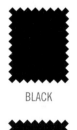
BLACK-BROWN

CHARCOAL

DARK NAVY

PEWTER

TAUPE

Now find out whether you are
Deep and Warm: **go to page 50** or
Deep and Cool: **go to page 54**.

# deep color palette

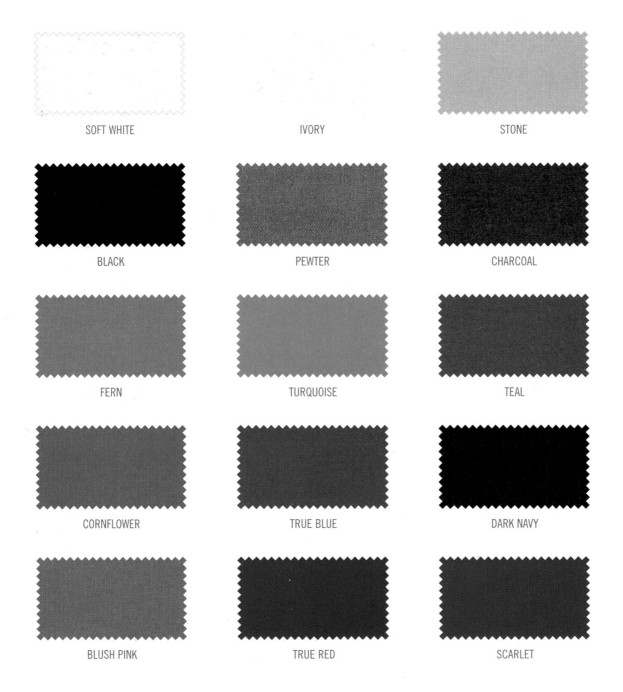

SOFT WHITE

IVORY

STONE

BLACK

PEWTER

CHARCOAL

FERN

TURQUOISE

TEAL

CORNFLOWER

TRUE BLUE

DARK NAVY

BLUSH PINK

TRUE RED

SCARLET

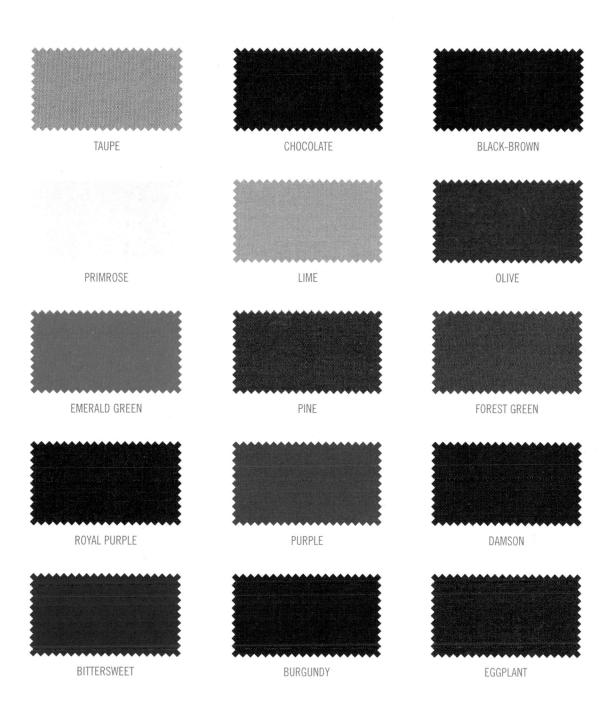

TAUPE

CHOCOLATE

BLACK-BROWN

PRIMROSE

LIME

OLIVE

EMERALD GREEN

PINE

FOREST GREEN

ROYAL PURPLE

PURPLE

DAMSON

BITTERSWEET

BURGUNDY

EGGPLANT

# deep & warm

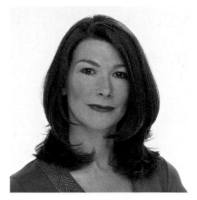

- Take a close look at your hair color. When in the sunlight or under a spotlight, do you see warm or red tones in your hair?
- Does your skin look golden, and do you have some freckles?
- Are your eyes more golden brown than ebony brown, perhaps with flecks of green or yellow in them?
- Do the color test with salmon and fuchsia, and with olive and dark teal: *go to page 33*. You should find that your best pink is salmon, a warm shade with some yellow in it, while the olive will suit you better than the dark teal.

Your secondary characteristic is warm. The softer, warmer (yellow) undertone of your additional colors will complement your look.

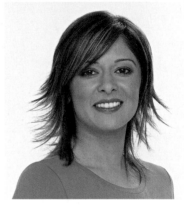

## your additional colors

As a Deep and Warm, you can now add these 12 extra shades to your master palette. Avoid wearing pale shades on their own and colors with an overall cool look. Charcoal, black, and dark navy look best on you when warmed up with camel, salmon, or terracotta.

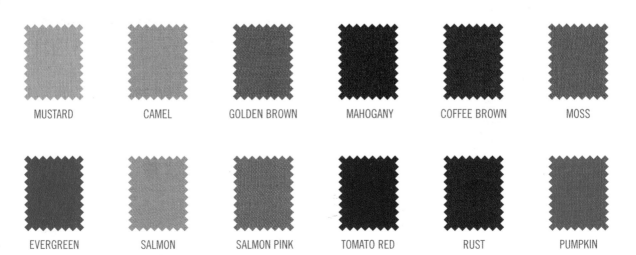

| MUSTARD | CAMEL | GOLDEN BROWN | MAHOGANY | COFFEE BROWN | MOSS |
|---|---|---|---|---|---|
| EVERGREEN | SALMON | SALMON PINK | TOMATO RED | RUST | PUMPKIN |

# in your makeup bag

**EYE PENCIL**   BROWN

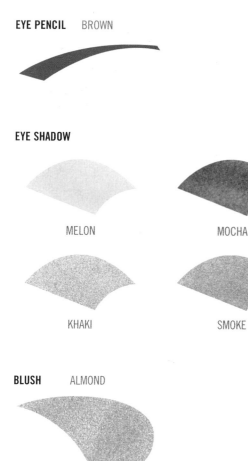

**EYE SHADOW**

MELON

MOCHA

KHAKI

SMOKE

**BLUSH**   ALMOND

**LIP PENCIL**   RUSSET

**LIPSTICK**   TOMATO

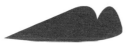

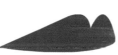

TERRACOTTA

NUTMEG

## your face

- The overall look of your makeup should be dark and rich, with a warm undertone.
- For eye pencils try olive, brown, or eggplant.
- Accent eye shadows such as khaki, smoke, mocha, or other shades of brown will blend perfectly with melon, apricot, or fawn.
- Your blush will need some depth to it, so try warm almond.
- Darker shades of lip pencil like russet or terracotta work best on you.
- Balance the richness of your complexion with lipstick shades like tomato, nutmeg, or terracotta; if you prefer a softer color, you will need to make sure that your eyes have a strong look for balance.

## your hair

- Since your hair is dark, natural highlights—gray or white—will often start to show earlier than you expect, so don't be afraid to use permanent or semipermanent tints.
- When adding color to your hair, the key is to match the color of your eyebrows to ensure that your hair is in harmony with the rest of your look.
- Add red and copper tones to enhance your hair's natural warmth.

# mixing colors with confidence deep & warm

## warm-weather combinations

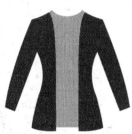

**BUSINESS WEAR**
coffee + mustard
golden brown + salmon
camel + tomato red
pewter + pumpkin

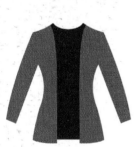

**CASUAL WEAR**
blush pink + bittersweet
fern + rust
taupe + olive
turquoise + salmon pink

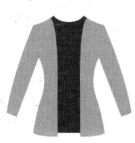

**SPECIAL OCCASION WEAR**
lime + olive
salmon + pumpkin
mustard + primrose
tomato red + salmon pink

## cool-weather combinations

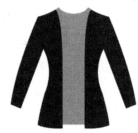

**BUSINESS WEAR**
eggplant + salmon
black-brown + salmon pink
pine + camel
royal purple + golden brown

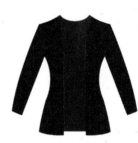

**CASUAL WEAR**
chocolate + bittersweet
olive + scarlet
purple + camel
mahogany + moss

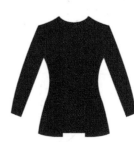

**SPECIAL OCCASION WEAR**
true red + rust
forest + evergreen
burgundy + mahogany
damson + olive

**LEFT** *Forest green is a great color for someone who is Deep and Warm.*

## ALTERNATIVE TO BLACK

Black is wonderful on you—it balances your deep, rich coloring. As an alternative, and to add a little individuality to your look, you can bring in the other dark shades of your palette such as the browns, but also think of choosing some of your dark greens such as olive and forest. For something a little more colorful, try the warm damson, burgundy, and eggplant from your palette. As a Deep, you can wear two dark colors together or wear a lighter shade with your dark neutral colors, bringing this in with accessories, if you prefer. However, in the summertime, you might like to wear lighter pewters and taupes instead of black, so add tomato red, pumpkin, or rust.

Now that you know your color palette, find out how to reflect your style through color: **go to pages 144–161.**

# deep & cool

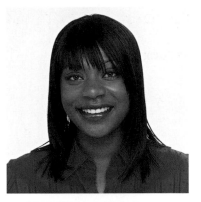

- Take a close look at your hair color in good light. Does it have an ebony tone?
- Do you have either porcelain skin or olive or black skin with a slight blue tinge?
- Are your eyes dark brown or ebony?
- Do the color test with salmon pink and fuchsia, and with olive and teal: *go to page 33*. You should find that your best pink is the cool fuchsia, while the dark teal will suit you better than the olive.

Your secondary characteristic is cool. Notice that there is a blue undertone and a clarity to your additional colors, which will complement your cool coloring.

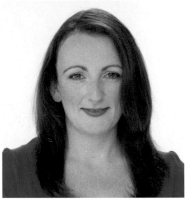

## your additional colors

As a Deep and Cool, you can now add these 12 extra shades to your master palette. Avoid very warm shades and colors with a strong yellow undertone. When you wear lime, olive, or bittersweet, balance them with royal purple, dark navy, or pine.

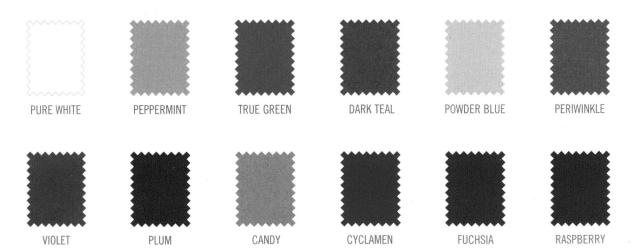

| PURE WHITE | PEPPERMINT | TRUE GREEN | DARK TEAL | POWDER BLUE | PERIWINKLE |
| VIOLET | PLUM | CANDY | CYCLAMEN | FUCHSIA | RASPBERRY |

# in your makeup bag

**EYE PENCIL**    EGGPLANT

**EYE SHADOW**

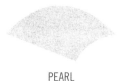

PEARL

SMOKE

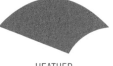

HEATHER

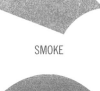

STEEL

**BLUSH**    PORT

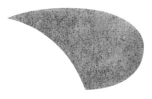

**LIP PENCIL**  RED

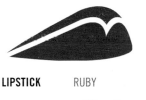

**LIPSTICK**     RUBY

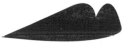

FIESTA

SOFT MAUVE

# your face

- The overall look of your makeup should be dark and rich, with a cool undertone.
- For eye pencils try eggplant, granite, or dark blue.
- Accent eye shadows such as heather, blue, smoke, steel, and other shades of gray will blend perfectly with pearl or pale pink.
- Your blush will need some depth to it, so try cool and deep tones like port.
- Darker shades of lip pencil work best: try red or rose.
- Balance your look with bold lipsticks such as ruby, fiesta or soft mauve. If you prefer to wear a softer color, you will need to make sure that your eyes have a strong look for balance.

# your hair

- Natural highlights tend to appear earlier in dark hair, but going gray will look stunning on you—though your dominant coloring may become cool.
- Don't be afraid to add color using permanent or semipermanent tints. Be guided by the natural color of your eyebrows to make sure that your hair is in harmony with the rest of your look.
- Use plummy shades to enhance the cool tones of your hair; avoid red and copper.

# mixing colors with confidence deep & cool

## warm-weather combinations

## cool-weather combinations

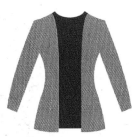

### BUSINESS WEAR

pewter + fuchsia
teal + peppermint
true blue + pure white
raspberry + ivory

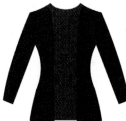

### BUSINESS WEAR

black + chocolate
dark navy + dark teal
black-brown + plum
forest + true green

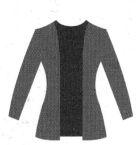

### CASUAL WEAR

cornflower + cyclamen
turquoise + violet
lime + true green
blush pink + raspberry

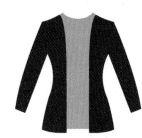

### CASUAL WEAR

damson + peppermint
raspberry + black
emerald green + violet
burgundy + cyclamen

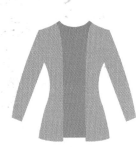

### SPECIAL OCCASION WEAR

peppermint + turquoise
periwinkle + royal purple
scarlet + plum
true blue + powder blue

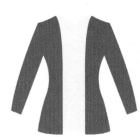

### SPECIAL OCCASION WEAR

true green + soft white
damson + violet
cyclamen + blush pink
black + lime

**LEFT** *Plum and cyclamen worn together make a perfect combination for someone who is Deep and Cool.*

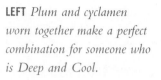

## ALTERNATIVE TO BLACK

Black is a major part of your wardrobe and will look good worn on its own or with another dark color. Because of your deep and cool coloring, shades of eggplant and purple are stunning against your skin. They can be worn on their own or combined with contrasting fuchsias or dark teals for a more dramatic look. In the evening, instead of a classic little black dress, you might want to wear a striking outfit in raspberry, true green, or violet for maximum impact. In the summertime, mix your lighter neutrals with dark, strong tones. If you wear pure white, accessorize with jewelry or scarves in bolder colors.

Now that you know your color palette, find out how to reflect your style through color: **go to pages 144–161**.

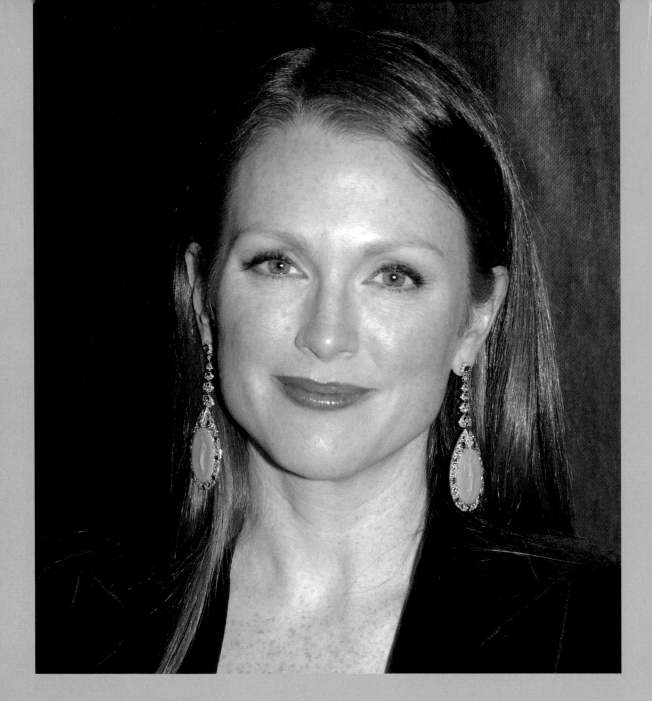

# warm

American actress Julianne Moore has the russet-colored hair and creamy porcelain skin of a classic Warm.

# are you a warm?

## do you have...

- red-toned hair in any shade from strawberry blonde to auburn?
- green, brown, or blue eyes?
- eyebrows in a warm tone, from reddish to brown?
- reddish or blonde eyelashes?
- porcelain skin, possibly with an abundance of freckles, or darker-toned skin with a golden glow to it?

## your look is

- Warm and golden.
- The undertone of your skin is warm.
- Your overall look is medium in depth.
- You may be either clear or soft.

## your ideal colors

For a master color palette: *go to pages 60–61*.

## how to wear your colors

Because your overall look is warm, the golden rule is to balance it by choosing colors that have a warm (yellow) undertone. You will always look best in colors that are medium in depth, rather than light or deep. When wearing navy or gray, warm them up with tones of yellow, salmon, or peach.

## be careful

Your look is warm and golden, so don't be tempted to buy items in baby pink or icy violet, because these colors will make you look gray. When wearing the darker neutrals in your palette, try to balance them with the lighter or paler shades—your overall look should be medium in depth. Keep makeup colors warm, especially blush and lipstick. Salmon and peachy shades will make you come alive. Avoid black mascara and eyeliner.

## investment buys

The following colors are ideal choices for items that you plan to keep for a long time. These shades will complement the majority of your other colors:

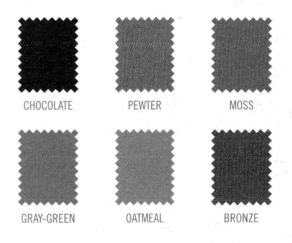

| CHOCOLATE | PEWTER | MOSS |
| --- | --- | --- |
| GRAY-GREEN | OATMEAL | BRONZE |

Now find out whether you are
Warm and Soft: **go to page 62** or
Warm and Clear: **go to page 66**.

# warm color palette

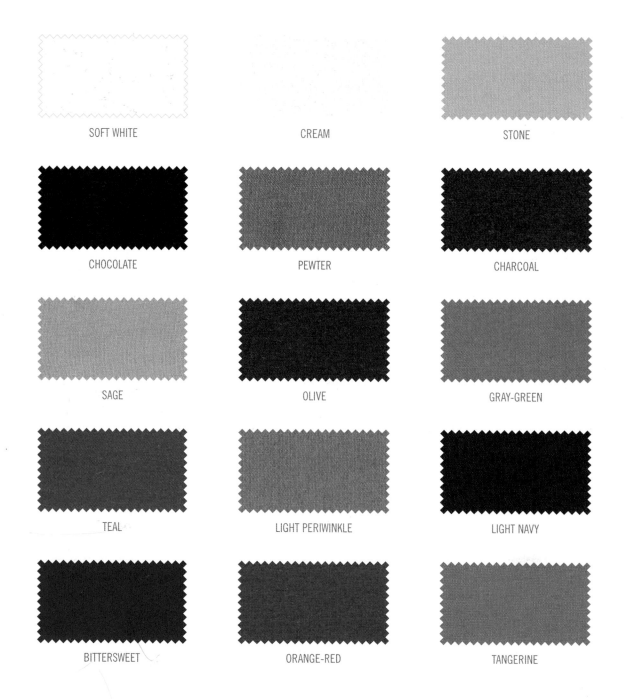

| | | |
|---|---|---|
| SOFT WHITE | CREAM | STONE |
| CHOCOLATE | PEWTER | CHARCOAL |
| SAGE | OLIVE | GRAY-GREEN |
| TEAL | LIGHT PERIWINKLE | LIGHT NAVY |
| BITTERSWEET | ORANGE-RED | TANGERINE |

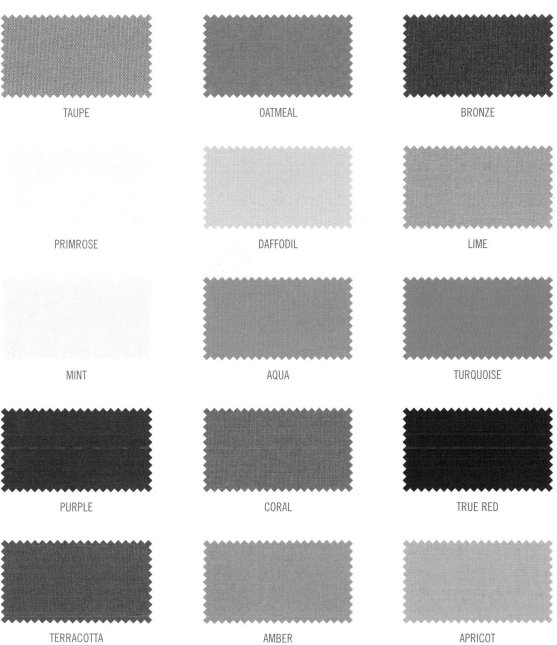

TAUPE

OATMEAL

BRONZE

PRIMROSE

DAFFODIL

LIME

MINT

AQUA

TURQUOISE

PURPLE

CORAL

TRUE RED

TERRACOTTA

AMBER

APRICOT

# warm & soft

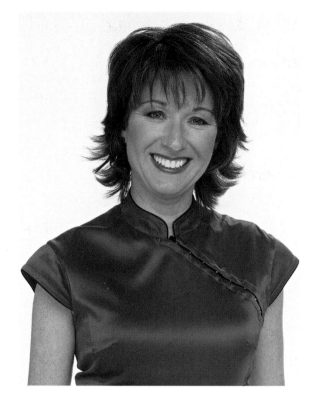

- Take a close look at your hair color. Would you describe it as auburn?
- Does your skin tone have a richness to it?
- Do you have brown or topaz-colored eyes?
- Do the color test with pumpkin and light peach, and then with light moss and olive: *go to page 33*. You should find that the deeper shades suit you better than the paler ones. Your best orange will be pumpkin, while the olive will suit you better than the light moss.

Your secondary characteristic is soft. Your additional colors will add depth and a softness to your main palette.

## your additional colors

As a Warm and Soft, you can now add these 12 extra shades to your master color palette. The charcoal and light navy in your master palette can be warmed up with salmon, mustard, or tomato red. Coffee brown, mahogany, and evergreen are also great neutrals.

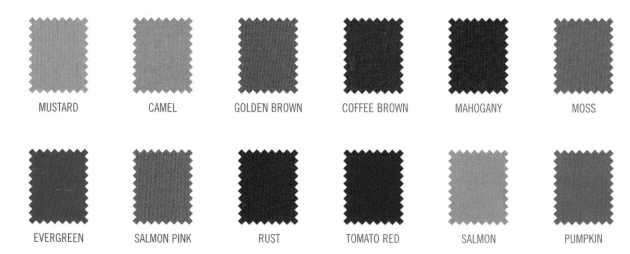

| MUSTARD | CAMEL | GOLDEN BROWN | COFFEE BROWN | MAHOGANY | MOSS |
| EVERGREEN | SALMON PINK | RUST | TOMATO RED | SALMON | PUMPKIN |

# in your makeup bag

**EYE PENCIL**   MOSS

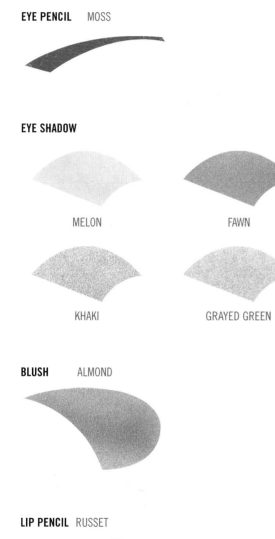

**EYE SHADOW**

MELON

FAWN

KHAKI

GRAYED GREEN

**BLUSH**   ALMOND

**LIP PENCIL**  RUSSET

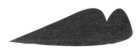

**LIPSTICK**   TERRACOTTA

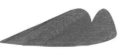

MAHOGANY

COPPER

# your face

- The overall look of your makeup should be warm and rich in order to enhance your golden coloring.
- For eye pencils try moss or brown.
- Accent eye shadows such as grayed green or khaki will blend well with fawn or melon, while shades of brown and tangerine will blend with apricot.
- Your blush will need to be warm and golden, so try almond or salmon.
- Warm shades of lip pencil work best on you: try russet or spicy browns.
- Balance your whole look with golden shades of lipstick such as terracotta, copper, or mahogany.

# your hair

- Your hair will be dark auburn or brown, with many warm highlights in it. Add rich, warm gold or copper tones if you want to enhance the richness of the color.
- When natural gray highlights start to appear, cover them with a copper or red tint; don't be tempted to go any darker, or you will change your dominant coloring type.
- Remember, your dominant palette will also change if you leave the gray uncolored.

# mixing colors with confidence warm & soft

## warm-weather combinations

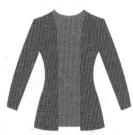

**BUSINESS WEAR**
golden brown + coral
moss + salmon
oatmeal + tomato red
gray-green + mustard

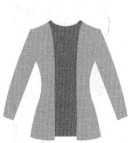

**CASUAL WEAR**
lime + salmon pink
orange-red + rust
stone + pumpkin
light periwinkle + camel

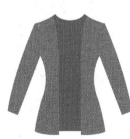

**SPECIAL OCCASION WEAR**
tangerine + pumpkin
moss + olive
tomato red + rust
apricot + salmon pink

## cool-weather combinations

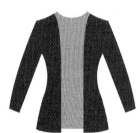

**BUSINESS WEAR**
olive + sage
chocolate + rust
charcoal + pumpkin
teal + salmon

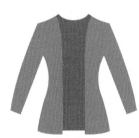

**CASUAL WEAR**
turquoise + pumpkin
rust + amber
evergreen + lime
terracotta + coffee brown

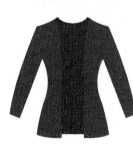

**SPECIAL OCCASION WEAR**
coffee brown + mahogany
bittersweet + tomato red
pumpkin + tangerine
purple + mahogany

**LEFT** *All shades of rust and terracotta give a stunning look for someone who is Warm and Soft.*

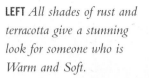

## ALTERNATIVE TO BLACK

Black is not in your palette; an excellent alternative is chocolate, which can be combined with most of the other colors in your palette. Depending on the occasion, you can think about wearing olives and bronzes, which again can be mixed with all your shades of reds, corals, and yellows to adapt them to business, casual, or special occasion wear. If you work in a formal environment, charcoal gray and navy may be more appropriate and will need to be warmed up with your yellows and corals. In hot climates, your oatmeals and camels are great alternatives to a dressed-up black, mixed with the turquoises and aquas.

Now that you know your color palette, find out how to reflect your style through color: **go to pages 144–161**.

# warm & clear

- Take a close look at your hair color. Is it more ginger or strawberry blonde than auburn?
- Do you have porcelain skin that may be sensitive to the sun?
- Are your eyes bright blue or green?
- Do the color test with pumpkin and light peach, and then with light moss and olive: *go to page 33*. You should find that your best shades are the paler, less intense ones—light peach will suit you better than pumpkin, and the light moss will enhance your coloring more than the olive.

Your secondary characteristic is clear. Notice that your additional shades have a lightness and a clarity to them.

## your additional colors

As a Warm and Clear, you can now add these 12 extra shades to your master palette. Warm up light navy and charcoal with yellow-green, peach, or light gold. Chocolate will need to be contrasted with a lighter shade like coral pink, light moss, or buttermilk.

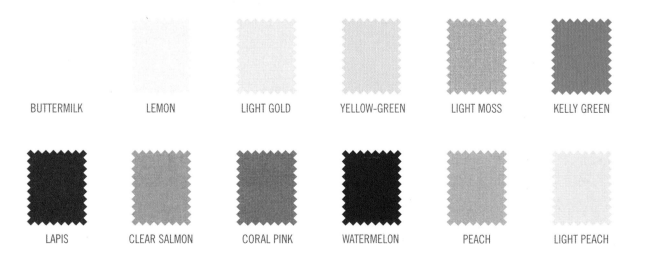

| BUTTERMILK | LEMON | LIGHT GOLD | YELLOW-GREEN | LIGHT MOSS | KELLY GREEN |
|---|---|---|---|---|---|
| LAPIS | CLEAR SALMON | CORAL PINK | WATERMELON | PEACH | LIGHT PEACH |

# in your makeup bag

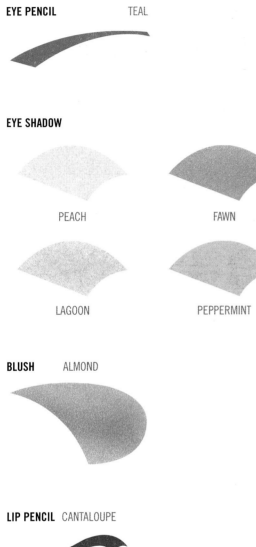

**EYE PENCIL**    TEAL

**EYE SHADOW**

PEACH

FAWN

LAGOON

PEPPERMINT

**BLUSH**    ALMOND

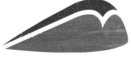

**LIP PENCIL**  CANTALOUPE

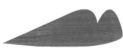

**LIPSTICK**    CORAL

TULIP

TOPAZ

# your face

- The overall look of your makeup should be warm, bright, and clear to enhance your coloring effectively.
- For eye pencils try teal, moss green, or coffee.
- Accent eye shadows such as peppermint or lagoon will blend perfectly with peach, fawn, shimmery gold, and cream.
- Your blush will need some warmth to it, so try almond or salmon.
- Bright, warm shades of lip pencil such as cantaloupe or coral will work best on you.
- Balance your whole look with lipstick in shades of coral, tulip, or topaz.

# your hair

- The light golden tones of your hair will naturally complement your golden skin tones, so make sure you keep your hair in peak condition to enhance the natural shine. If you want to add color, copper or strawberry highlights will work best.
- Use a golden tint when the natural gray highlights start to appear. Don't be tempted to go darker, or you will change your dominant coloring type.

# mixing colors with confidence warm & clear

## warm-weather combinations

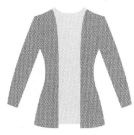

**BUSINESS WEAR**
taupe + yellow-green
bronze + light peach
oatmeal + clear salmon
light navy + peach

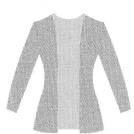

**CASUAL WEAR**
light moss + daffodil
aqua + lapis
orange-red + peach
stone + kelly green

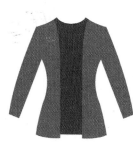

**SPECIAL OCCASION WEAR**
periwinkle + lapis
tangerine + peach
coral pink + coral
light moss + lime

## cool-weather combinations

**BUSINESS WEAR**
teal + buttermilk
chocolate + peach
charcoal + coral pink
pewter + light gold

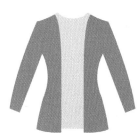

**CASUAL WEAR**
turquoise + yellow-green
amber + light peach
true red + lapis
moss + light gold

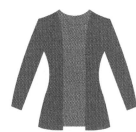

**SPECIAL OCCASION WEAR**
terracotta + coral pink
tomato red +
watermelon
purple + periwinkle
lapis + mint

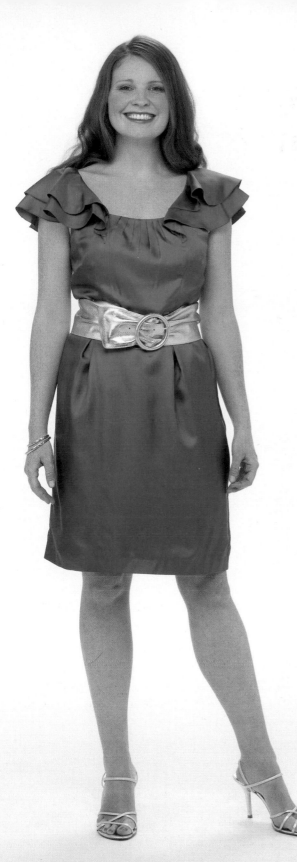

**LEFT** *Kelly green is a perfect color for someone with Warm and Clear coloring.*

## ALTERNATIVE TO BLACK

Many women with your Warm and Clear coloring feel they can wear black, but there are several alternatives, which are much more flattering and suitable for all occasions. Bronze and dark brown are great together, and teamed with pale yellow make a stylish substitute for black. If you have a formal business dress code, don't forget to warm up your charcoal and navy with peaches, corals, and even warm reds.

Now that you know your color palette, find out how to reflect your style through color: **go to pages 144–161**

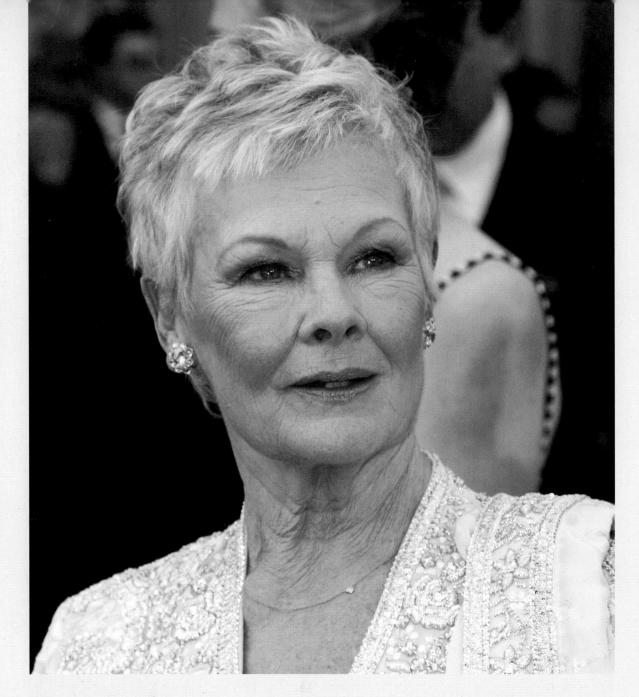

# cool

Oscar-winning British actress Judi Dench, with her distinctive gray cropped hair, has all the attributes of a Cool palette.

# are you a cool?

## do you have...

- ash tones in your hair, whether it is dark brown, blonde, white, or gray?
- gray, blue, green, or clear brown eyes?
- eyebrows and eyelashes that range in color from the lighter shade of blonde to dark brown?
- pink undertones to your skin? A black or brown skin may have a slight blue tinge.

## your look is

- Cool and pinkish.
- The undertone of your skin is cool.
- The overall depth of your coloring is medium to deep.
- The clarity of your look may be either clear or soft.

## your ideal colors

For a master color palette: *go to pages 72–73*.

## how to wear your colors

Because your look is cool and pinkish, all your colors need to have a cool (blue) undertone, preferably with some contrast. You will always look best in medium to deep colors. If you wear brown, balance it with cool shades from your palette, such as teal or rose pink.

## be careful

Avoid colors that have a warm, yellow tone, because they will make your skin appear sallow. If you do wear yellow, it must be an icy lemon. Browns need to have a pinky, rather than yellow, tone. When wearing your darker neutrals, balance them with the lighter and brighter shades from your color chart and avoid wearing two dark neutrals together. Keep all your makeup colors cool, and beware of brown-based lipsticks, especially pale, natural-looking shades.

## investment buys

When buying items with longevity, these shades are the ideal choices and will complement most of the other colors in your cool palette:

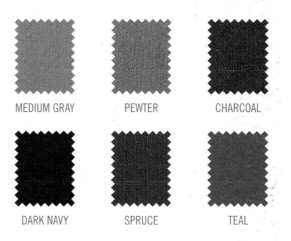

| MEDIUM GRAY | PEWTER | CHARCOAL |
| DARK NAVY | SPRUCE | TEAL |

Now find out whether you are
Cool and Soft: **go to page 74** or
Cool and Clear: **go to page 78**.

# cool color palette

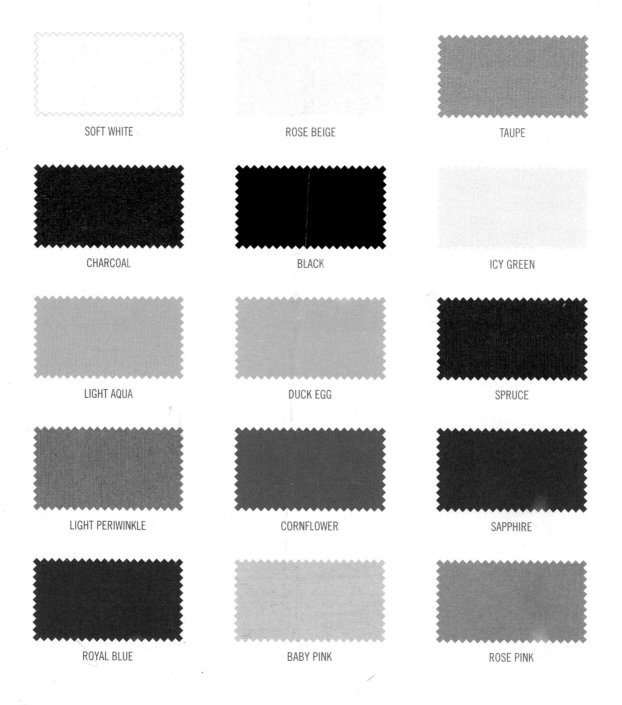

SOFT WHITE

ROSE BEIGE

TAUPE

CHARCOAL

BLACK

ICY GREEN

LIGHT AQUA

DUCK EGG

SPRUCE

LIGHT PERIWINKLE

CORNFLOWER

SAPPHIRE

ROYAL BLUE

BABY PINK

ROSE PINK

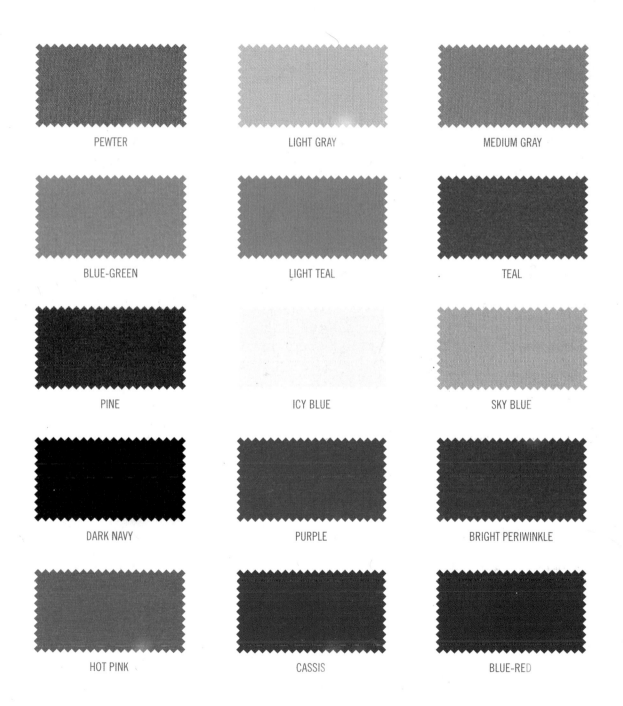

PEWTER

LIGHT GRAY

MEDIUM GRAY

BLUE-GREEN

LIGHT TEAL

TEAL

PINE

ICY BLUE

SKY BLUE

DARK NAVY

PURPLE

BRIGHT PERIWINKLE

HOT PINK

CASSIS

BLUE-RED

# cool & soft

- Take a close look at your hair color, either in natural sunlight or under a spotlight. Does it have ash tones?
- Does your skin tone have a softness to it?
- Are your eyes light blue or green?
- Do the color test with lavender and fuchsia, and then with amethyst and plum: *go to page 33*. You should find that you look best in the softer shades of lavender and amethyst, rather than the stronger fuchsia and plum.

Your secondary characteristic is soft. Your additional colors will add a lightness and softness to your main palette that will complement your cool coloring.

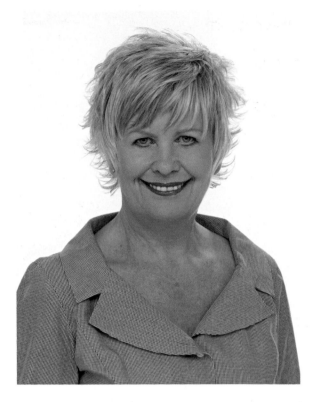

## your additional colors

As a Cool and Soft, you can now add these 12 extra shades to your master palette. When you are wearing black, soften the look by using soft, pale colors such as bluebell, powder pink, or eau de nil near your face. Think about the type of fabrics you'll wear. Tweeds are great.

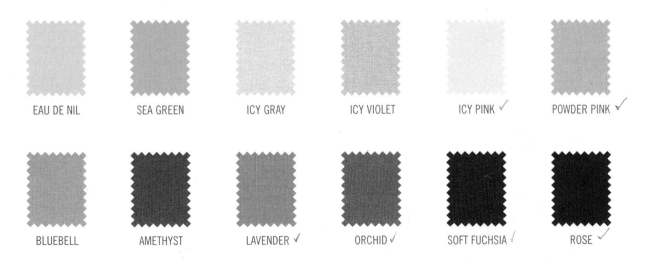

| EAU DE NIL | SEA GREEN | ICY GRAY | ICY VIOLET | ICY PINK ✓ | POWDER PINK ✓ |
| BLUEBELL | AMETHYST | LAVENDER ✓ | ORCHID ✓ | SOFT FUCHSIA ✓ | ROSE ✓ |

## in your makeup bag

**EYE PENCIL**   AMETHYST

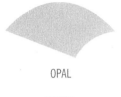

**EYE SHADOW**

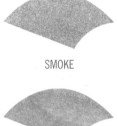

OPAL

SMOKE

HEATHER

LILAC

**BLUSH**   CANDY

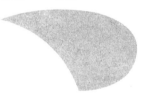

**LIP PENCIL**   ROSE

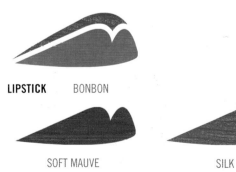

**LIPSTICK**   BONBON

SOFT MAUVE

SILK

## your face

- The overall look of your makeup should be cool, using blue-based shades to balance your dominant coloring.
- For eye pencils try amethyst or granite.
- Accent eye shadows such as heather, smoke, and gray-blue shades will work well with opal, lilac, or pewter grays.
- Your blush will need cool pink undertones; candy or rose will suit you.
- Cool, soft shades of lip pencil work best: try rose or pink.
- Balance your whole look with lipstick in all shades of cool pinks and mauves such as bonbon, soft mauve, silk, or soft berry shades.

## your hair

- Your hair will be dark blonde to light brown or a soft, silvery gray.
- The ash tones in your hair mean that you have the advantage of graying gracefully, but you may find that you need to add a little more color to your look by using brighter makeup or by wearing colors with more contrast.
- If you decide to color your hair, be sure to use platinum or ash tones, and avoid red tints.

# mixing colors with confidence cool & soft

## warm-weather combinations

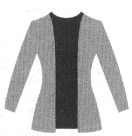

**BUSINESS WEAR**

taupe + rose
medium gray + icy violet
sapphire + powder pink
light periwinkle +
lavender

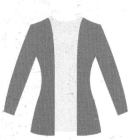

**CASUAL WEAR**

light teal + icy pink
orchid + aqua
duck egg + icy gray
cornflower + eau de nil

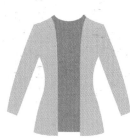

**SPECIAL OCCASION WEAR**

sea green + blue-green
amethyst + icy violet
rose pink + powder pink
bluebell + sky blue

## cool-weather combinations

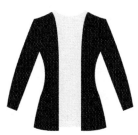

**BUSINESS WEAR**

dark navy + icy pink
charcoal + orchid
pewter + lavender
sapphire + bluebell

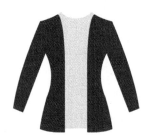

**CASUAL WEAR**

royal blue + icy gray
rose + pastel pink
teal + soft fuchsia
purple + icy violet

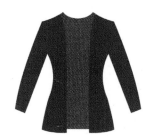

**SPECIAL OCCASION WEAR**

cassis + soft fuchsia
blue-red + rose
aqua + eau de nil
bright periwinkle + amethyst

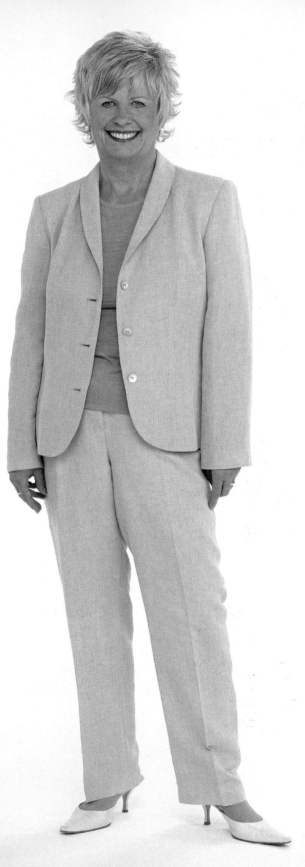

**LEFT** *Two contrasting shades of turquoise make a great combination for someone who is Cool and Soft.*

## ALTERNATIVE TO BLACK

Although black is in your palette, charcoal is a great alternative, particularly in a soft fabric like a washed silk, tweed, or velvet. Team rose, amethyst, or powder pink with your charcoal gray for a flattering look. When wearing your taupes and pewters, try them with the aquas and teals from your palette. Dark navy will always be a staple in your wardrobe, and if you are daring enough, try some red, too, either as a flash from a belt or scarf, or as an outfit on its own. For evening looks, nothing will be more elegant than your purples and periwinkles lifted with pearls, diamonds, or silver jewelry.

Now that you know your color palette, find out how to reflect your style through color: **go to pages 144–161**

# cool & clear

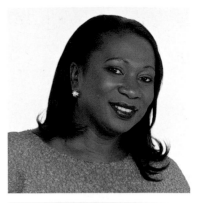

- Take a close look at your hair color under the light. If it is gray, is your hair more silver than ash? If you are dark-haired, is your hair really dark?
- Is there a clarity about your skin color?
- Are your eyes dark blue, green, or clear brown?
- Do the color test with lavender and fuchsia, and then with amethyst and plum: *go to page 33.* You should find that you look best in fuchsia and plum.

Your secondary characteristic is clear. Your additional colors include darker shades, and they will all add clarity to your main color palette.

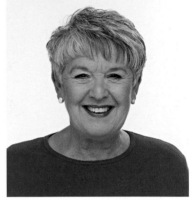

## your additional colors

As a Cool and Clear, you can now add these 12 extra shades to your main palette. When you wear taupe, pewter, or medium to light gray,

balance these lighter tones with clearer and deeper shades from your palette such as violet, true green, or raspberry.

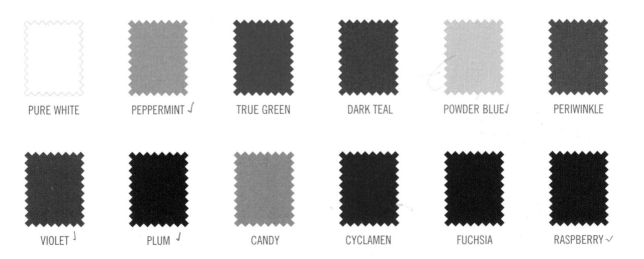

| PURE WHITE | PEPPERMINT ✓ | TRUE GREEN | DARK TEAL | POWDER BLUE ✓ | PERIWINKLE |
| VIOLET ✓ | PLUM ✓ | CANDY | CYCLAMEN | FUCHSIA | RASPBERRY ✓ |

# in your makeup bag

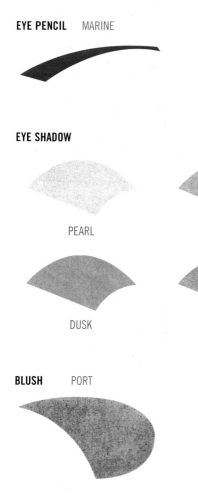

**EYE PENCIL**  MARINE

**EYE SHADOW**

PEARL

COCOA

DUSK

DELPH

**BLUSH**  PORT

**LIP PENCIL**  POSIE

**LIPSTICK**  CERISE

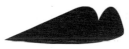

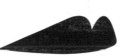

RUBY

FIESTA

## your face

- The overall look of your makeup should be cool, using cool shades to balance your dominant coloring.
- For eye pencils try marine, soft black, or violet-blue.
- Accent eye shadows such as cocoa, delph, and shades of dark, smoky grays will blend well with pearl, dusk, or aqua.
- Your blush will need to be cool, so try a shade like port.
- Cool shades of lip pencil like posie work best for you.
- Balance your whole look with cool, clear lipstick colors like cerise, fiesta, or ruby.

## your hair

- You have dark brown or even black hair, with no apparent warmth to it. The strong colors in your palette work wonderfully with the striking cool tones of your hair.
- Use contrast in your makeup and clothes to balance your hair color.
- When your hair eventually turns gray, it will be a stunning pure white or silver gray.

# mixing colors with confidence cool & clear

## warm-weather combinations

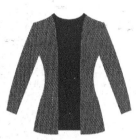

**BUSINESS WEAR**
pewter + fuchsia
charcoal + duck egg
periwinkle + icy blue
raspberry + pastel pink

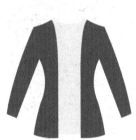

**CASUAL WEAR**
true green + icy green
royal blue + powder blue
violet + cassis
aqua + dark teal

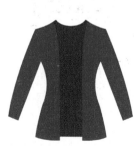

**SPECIAL OCCASION WEAR**
cyclamen + cassis
raspberry + plum
peppermint + spruce
light gray + black

## cool-weather combinations

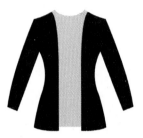

**BUSINESS WEAR**
black + powder blue
pine + peppermint
dark navy + true green
blue-red + pure white

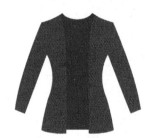

**CASUAL WEAR**
purple + fuchsia
raspberry + spruce
periwinkle + icy blue
charcoal + cyclamen

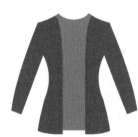

**SPECIAL OCCASION WEAR**
dark teal + light teal
plum + cyclamen
royal blue + powder blue
black + pure white

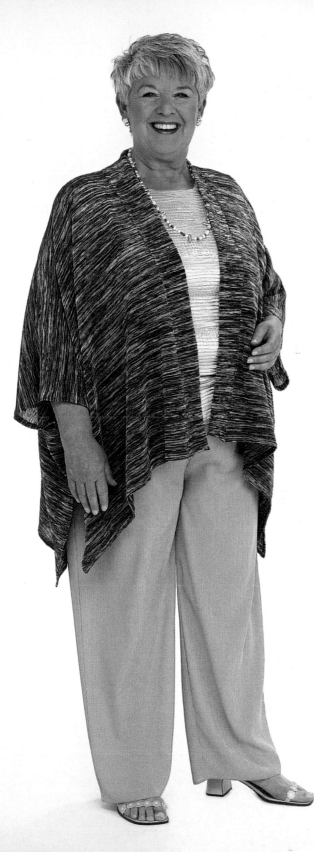

**LEFT** *The sheen of the silver fabric lifts your Cool and Clear look.*

## ALTERNATIVE TO BLACK

Although black is in your palette, there are many great alternatives that will look stunning with your coloring. Try royal blue with navy; the brightness of the royal blue gives you the contrast against the navy that you need. Don't forget that you will also look great in grays and dark greens, but team them with brightly colored jewels or a contrasting scarf. Remember that the lighter neutrals in your palette will look great with the really bright, contrasting shades.

Now that you know your color palette, find out how to reflect your style through color: **go to pages 144–161.**

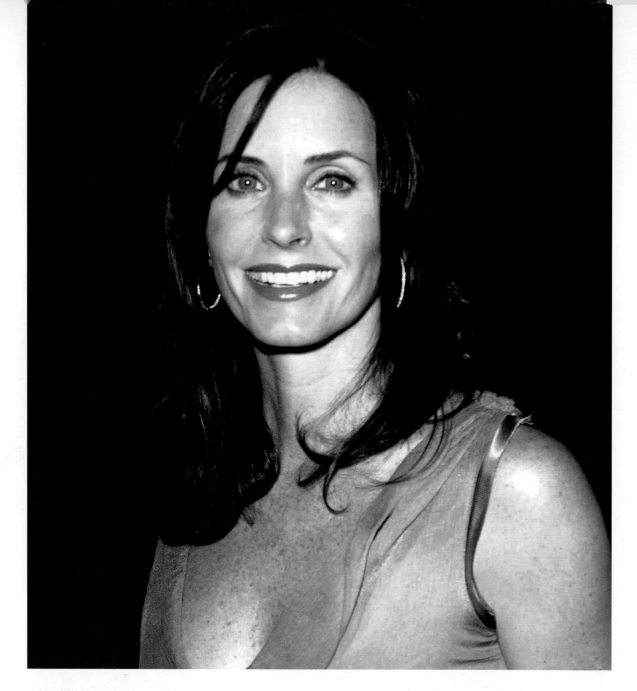

# clear

Star of the TV series
Friends, *Courtney
Cox Arquette is a perfect
example of someone
classified as a Clear.*

# are you a clear?

## do you have...
- dark hair?
- bright eyes that are your most striking feature, whether they are blue, green, or topaz? If you are dark-skinned there will be a noticeable contrast between the white of your eyes and the color of the iris.
- dark eyebrows and eyelashes?
- skin that can be any tone from light to dark?

## your look is
- Fresh and clear.
- The undertone of your skin may be either warm or cool.
- Your overall look is contrasting between light and dark.
- You have a decidedly clear look.

## your ideal colors
For a master color palette: *go to pages 84–85*.

## how to wear your colors
Because your look is contrasting (for example, dark hair, bright eyes and, if Caucasian, porcelain skin), you need to wear your colors in a way that balances this. You will always look good in a contrast of light and dark colors. If you wear sludgy colors like taupe and pewter, liven them up with the brightest shades from your palette. If you dress in a single color, make sure it is one of the most vivid from your palette.

## be careful
Basic neutrals like black, charcoal, and black-brown are great staples in your wardrobe, but do wear them with the lighter shades from your palette. You may be tempted to wear white in summer, but combine it with a bright color like scarlet, or even black, to keep a light and dark contrast.

## investment buys
For you, the best colors for items that will have longevity in your wardrobe are:

BLACK

BLACK-BROWN

DARK NAVY

CHARCOAL

PURPLE

ROYAL BLUE

Now find out whether you are
Clear and Warm: **go to page 86** or
Clear and Cool: **go to page 90**.

# clear color palette

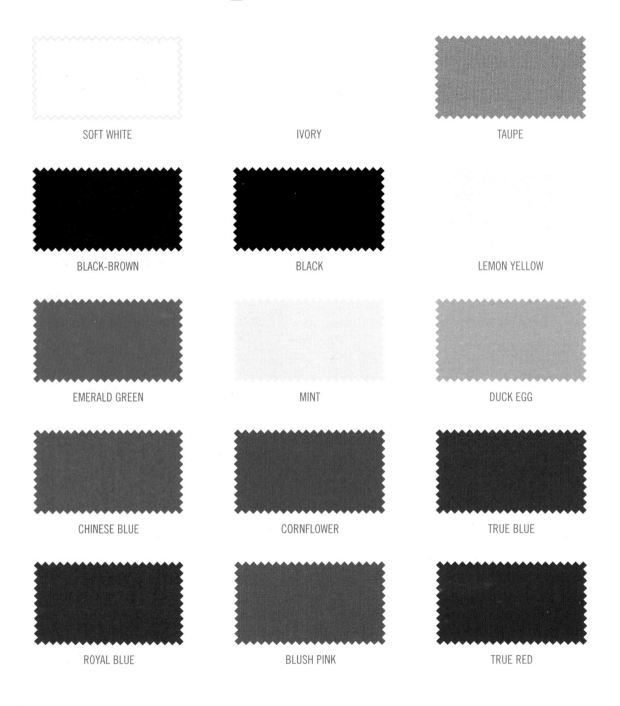

| | | |
|---|---|---|
| SOFT WHITE | IVORY | TAUPE |
| BLACK-BROWN | BLACK | LEMON YELLOW |
| EMERALD GREEN | MINT | DUCK EGG |
| CHINESE BLUE | CORNFLOWER | TRUE BLUE |
| ROYAL BLUE | BLUSH PINK | TRUE RED |

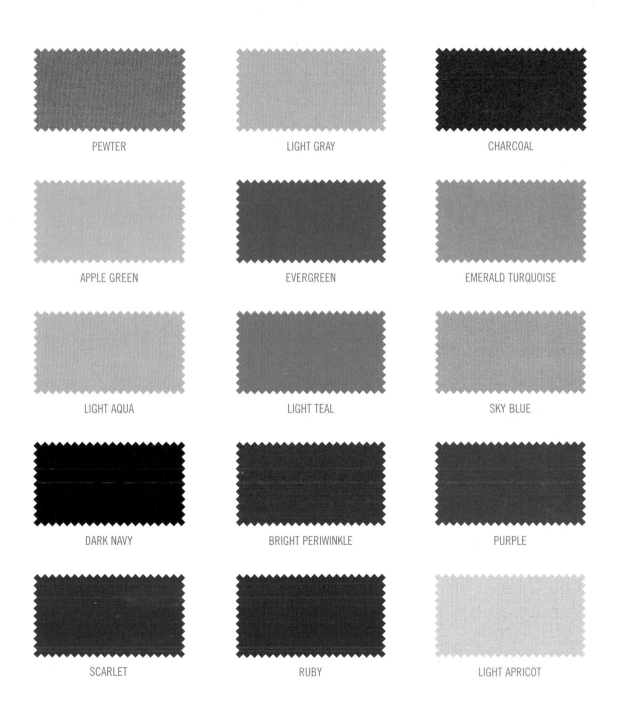

PEWTER

LIGHT GRAY

CHARCOAL

APPLE GREEN

EVERGREEN

EMERALD TURQUOISE

LIGHT AQUA

LIGHT TEAL

SKY BLUE

DARK NAVY

BRIGHT PERIWINKLE

PURPLE

SCARLET

RUBY

LIGHT APRICOT

# clear & warm

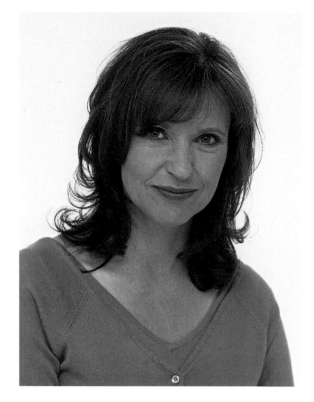

- Take a close look at your hair color under good light. Is it dark with warm highlights?
- Does your skin have warm, golden undertones and maybe a few freckles?
- Are your eyes clear bright blue, clear green, or clear topaz?
- Do the color test with clear salmon and cyclamen, and then with kelly green and dark teal: *go to page 33*. You should find that your best shade of pink is a clear salmon, while the kelly green will suit you better than the dark teal.

Your secondary characteristic is warm. Your additional colors all have warmth to them and include some lighter shades.

## your additional colors

As a Clear and Warm, you can add these 12 extra shades to your master palette. When you wear lighter tones like taupe, pewter, or medium to light gray, balance them with clearer, deeper shades from your palette such as coral pink, kelly green, or lapis.

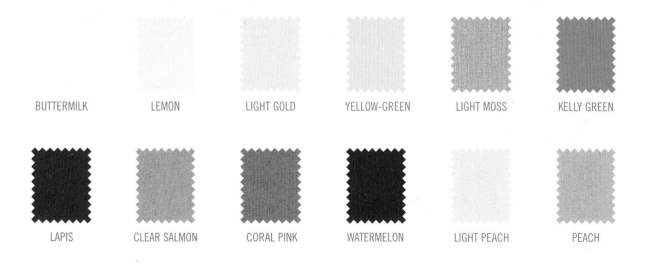

| BUTTERMILK | LEMON | LIGHT GOLD | YELLOW-GREEN | LIGHT MOSS | KELLY GREEN |

| LAPIS | CLEAR SALMON | CORAL PINK | WATERMELON | LIGHT PEACH | PEACH |

# in your makeup bag

**EYE PENCIL**  TEAL

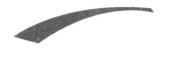

**EYE SHADOW**

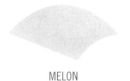

MELON

STEEL

PEPPERMINT

COCOA

**BLUSH**  SALMON

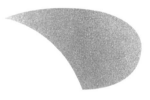

**LIP PENCIL**  CANTALOUPE

**LIPSTICK**  WARM PINK

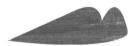

CORAL

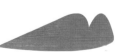

BREEZE

# your face

- The overall look of your makeup should be clear, and your contrasting look needs to be balanced with brighter colors. You may want to decide whether to emphasize either your eyes or your lips, but not both at once.
- For eye pencils try amethyst, violet-blue, or teal.
- Accent eye shadows like cocoa, steel, peppermint, or heather work well with either melon, peach, or apricot.
- Your blush will need some warmth to it, so a shade such as salmon is ideal.
- Brighter shades of lip pencil work best: try using cantaloupe.
- Balance your whole look with lipstick colors such as warm pink, coral, or breeze.

# your hair

- Your hair will be dark but with some golden or copper highlights. Keep the base color of your hair dark; don't be tempted to go blonde.
- If you want to add color, it is best to use varying colors of lowlights—two to three shades will enhance your natural color.
- Cover gray with a warm tint that will give the appearance of highlights. Gold or copper lowlights work well, as do warm, semipermanent tints.

# mixing colors with confidence clear & warm

## warm-weather combinations

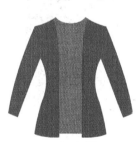

**BUSINESS WEAR**
pewter + yellow-green
sky blue + lapis
cornflower + light gold
emerald turquoise + light peach

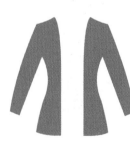

**CASUAL WEAR**
blush pink + coral pink
taupe + watermelon
true blue + buttermilk
apple green + yellow-green

**SPECIAL OCCASION WEAR**
light teal + buttermilk
Chinese blue + mint
coral pink + light apricot
bright periwinkle + light moss

## cool-weather combinations

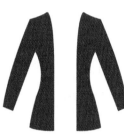

**BUSINESS WEAR**
lapis + ivory
black + clear salmon
charcoal + lemon
watermelon + light gray

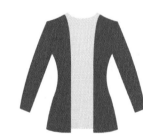

**CASUAL WEAR**
evergreen + yellow-green
purple + coral pink
royal blue + peach
black-brown + watermelon

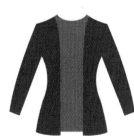

**SPECIAL OCCASION WEAR**
cornflower + lapis
light aqua + Chinese blue
ruby + clear salmon
emerald green + light moss

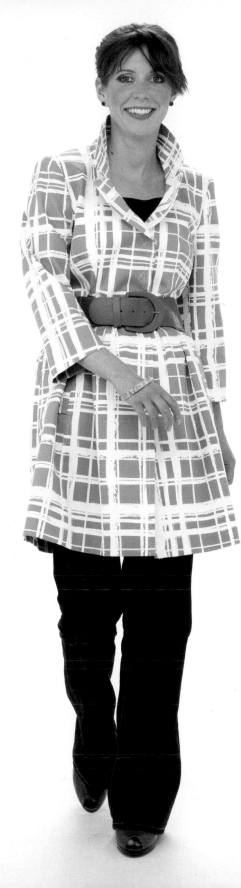

**LEFT** *Do not ignore the brighter colors from your palette for outerwear. Apple green and white make a fun combination.*

## ALTERNATIVE TO BLACK

Yes, you can wear black, but there are so many other shades that will be much more interesting on you. Purple is a color that has become increasingly popular over the past few years and can be found in the stores nearly every season. If wearing your grays and navys, try choosing them in a fabric with some sheen, such as silk, or adding some sparkle with stunning accessories, such as bold jewelry, bright shoes, or a beaded bag.

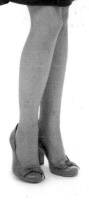

Now that you know your color palette, find out how to reflect your style through color: **go to pages 144–161**.

# clear & cool

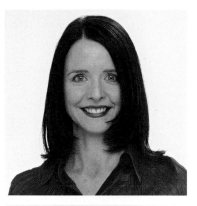

- Take a close look at your hair color in sunlight or under a spotlight. Does it have ebony tones?
- Does your porcelain skin have a pink tone to it? If you are black, does your skin have a coolness to it?
- Are your eyes dark green, blue, or clear brown?
- Do the color test with clear salmon and cyclamen, and then with kelly green and dark teal: *go to page 33*. You should find that your best shade of pink is cyclamen, while the dark teal will suit you better than the kelly green.

Your secondary characteristic is cool. Your additional colors will add coolness and depth to your main color palette.

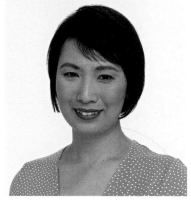

## your additional colors

As a Clear and Cool, you can now add these 12 extra shades to your master palette. When wearing the lighter shades of your palette, such as taupe and light gray, contrast them with ruby, bright periwinkle, emerald-turquoise, and turquoise. Do not forget to contrast your dark neutrals as well.

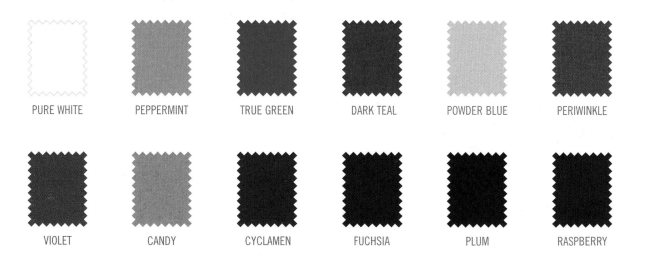

| PURE WHITE | PEPPERMINT | TRUE GREEN | DARK TEAL | POWDER BLUE | PERIWINKLE |
| VIOLET | CANDY | CYCLAMEN | FUCHSIA | PLUM | RASPBERRY |

# in your makeup bag

**EYE PENCIL**   MARINE

**EYE SHADOW**

CHAMPAGNE                    MERCURY

MOCHA                              PEWTER

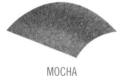

**BLUSH**   MARSALA

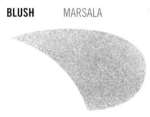

**LIP PENCIL**   RED

**LIPSTICK**   STRAWBERRY

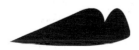

RUBY                              FIESTA

# your face

- The overall look of your makeup should be clear, and your contrasting look needs to be balanced with deeper colors.
- For eye pencils try dark blue or soft black.
- Accent eye shadows such as mercury, pewter, or mocha blended with champagne or smoky grays will look wonderful on you.
- Your blush needs to be cool and deep, so try shades like marsala.
- Darker shades of lip pencil like red or bright pink work best.
- Balance your whole look with lipstick colors such as strawberry, ruby, fiesta, or bright reds.

# your hair

- Your hair is dark brown or even black, and there will be a lack of warmth to it. If you have a dark or East Asian complexion, your hair may have a slight blue tinge.
- When adding color, use plummy (bluish) shades and avoid copper or red tones.
- When natural gray highlights start to appear, cover everything with a cool, plummy tint. If you decide to go with the gray, your basic palette may change to Cool and Clear (pages 78–81).

# mixing colors with confidence clear & cool

## warm-weather combinations

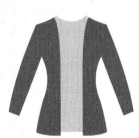

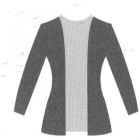

**BUSINESS WEAR**
pewter + cyclamen
true blue + powder blue
true red + pure white
peppermint + dark navy

**CASUAL WEAR**
periwinkle + light apricot
apple green + true green
scarlet + violet
dark teal + lemon yellow

**SPECIAL OCCASION WEAR**
Chinese blue + powder blue
violet + periwinkle
peppermint + mint
blush pink + raspberry

## cool-weather combinations

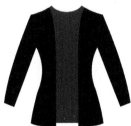

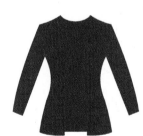

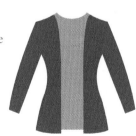

**BUSINESS WEAR**
black + ruby
true green + peppermint
navy + cyclamen
black-brown + violet

**CASUAL WEAR**
royal blue + fuchsia
bright periwinkle + violet
charcoal + cyclamen
blush pink + plum

**SPECIAL OCCASION WEAR**
evergreen + peppermint
dark teal + dark aqua
black + fuchsia
scarlet + violet

**LEFT** *A stylish dress in a bright pink is a stunning look for a Clear and Cool.*

## ALTERNATIVE TO BLACK

Contrast is a key element of your look, so here we have taken navy and white, and teamed them with sky blue for a different but professional look. Adding a contrasting-colored jacket to your basic navy pants or skirts is a fun way of introducing variety to your wardrobe. If you are wearing the lighter neutrals from your palette, remember to balance the look with a darker or brighter shade.

Now that you know your color palette, find out how to reflect your style through color: **go to pages 144–161.**

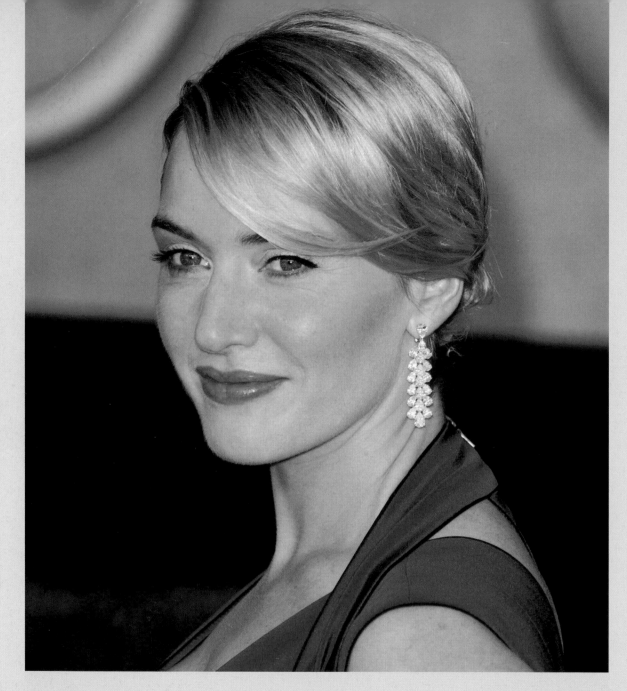

# soft

*With her highlighted hair and soft skin tone, British actress Kate Winslet is classified as a Soft.*

# are you a soft?

## do you have...
- dark blonde (mousy) or light brown hair?
- eyes that are a soft and muted color, whether blue, brown, hazel, or green, and that often change color?
- light to dark eyebrows and eyelashes?
- little contrast between the color of your hair, your eyes, and your skin, which may be any tone from light to dark?

## your look is
- Soft, with coloring characteristics that are apparently unrelated and may be confusing. You may have found a little of yourself in each of the previous five dominant coloring types, but you do not fit any of them exactly.
- The undertone of your skin may be either warm or cool.
- The overall depth of your coloring is medium.
- Your look is decidedly soft.

## your ideal colors
For a master color palette: *go to pages 96–97*.

## how to wear your colors
Because your look is blended, your colors need to be worn "tone on tone," with little contrast. You will always look best in tones of medium depth.

A monochromatic look suits you very well. If you wear the darker shades in your palette, balance them with colors that are only one or two tones lighter, and avoid high contrast.

## be careful
If you like to wear strong, bright colors, choose interesting combinations like sapphire and mint, purple and geranium, or damson and blush pink. Wear pale shades like soft white or shell with medium-depth colors rather than dark shades.

## investment buys
For you, the best colors for items that will have longevity in your wardrobe are:

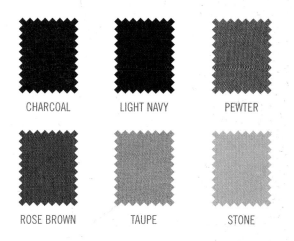

| CHARCOAL | LIGHT NAVY | PEWTER |
| ROSE BROWN | TAUPE | STONE |

Now find out whether you are
Soft and Warm: **go to page 98** or a
Soft and Cool: **go to page 102**.

# soft color palette

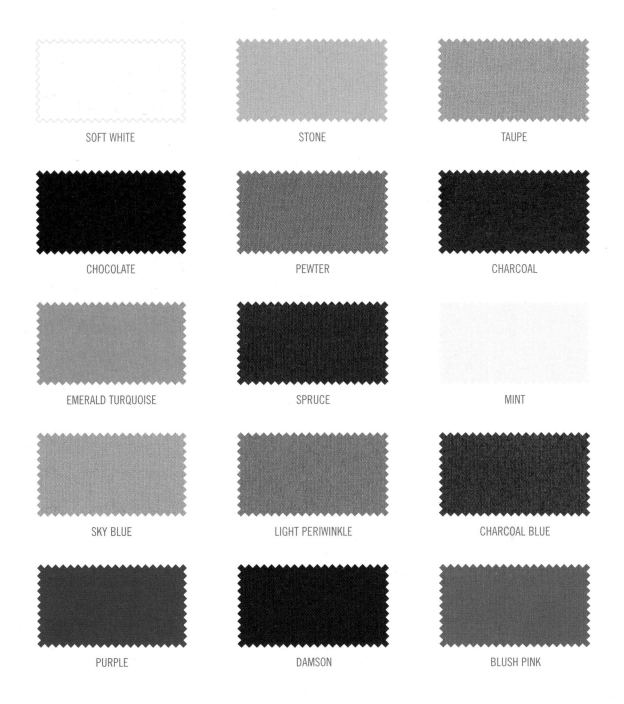

SOFT WHITE

STONE

TAUPE

CHOCOLATE

PEWTER

CHARCOAL

EMERALD TURQUOISE

SPRUCE

MINT

SKY BLUE

LIGHT PERIWINKLE

CHARCOAL BLUE

PURPLE

DAMSON

BLUSH PINK

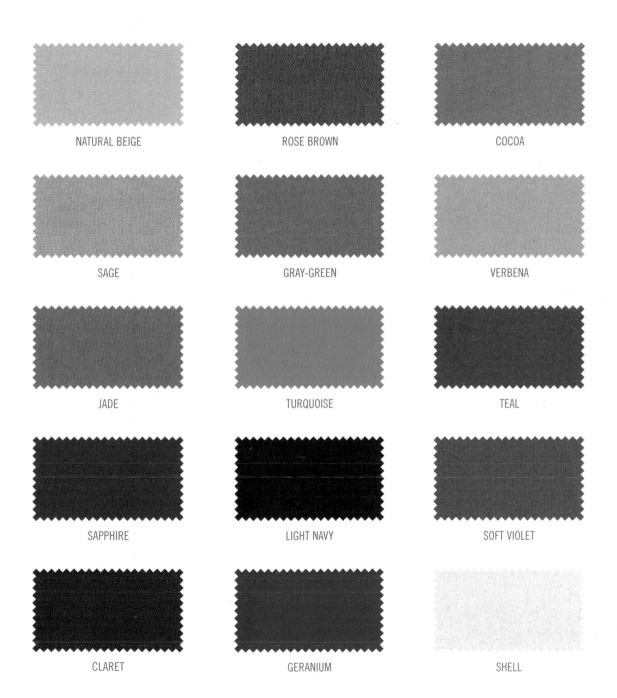

NATURAL BEIGE

ROSE BROWN

COCOA

SAGE

GRAY-GREEN

VERBENA

JADE

TURQUOISE

TEAL

SAPPHIRE

LIGHT NAVY

SOFT VIOLET

CLARET

GERANIUM

SHELL

# soft & warm

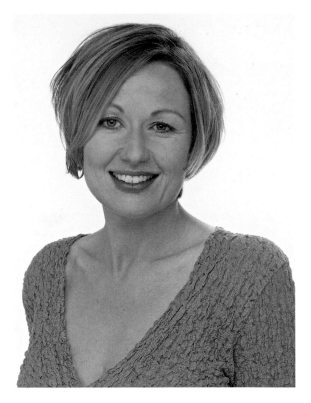

- Take a close look at your hair color. Is it golden blonde or light warm brown?
- Does your skin have golden undertones and maybe a few freckles as well?
- Are your eyes soft brown or soft hazel/moss?
- Do the color test with orchid and peach, and then with sea green and olive: **go to page 33.** You should find that your best shade of pink is peach, while olive tones will suit you better than cooler, blue-based sea greens.

Your secondary characteristic is warm. You will notice that all your additional colors have a warmth to them.

## your additional colors

As a Soft and Warm, you can now add these 12 extra shades to your master palette. Mix darker colors with a similar color, but one or two tones lighter—for example, wear light charcoal with moss, chocolate with golden brown or light navy with salmon.

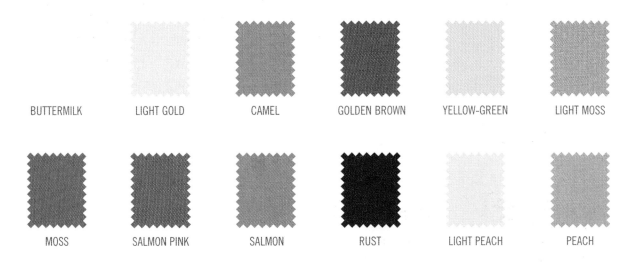

| BUTTERMILK | LIGHT GOLD | CAMEL | GOLDEN BROWN | YELLOW-GREEN | LIGHT MOSS |
| --- | --- | --- | --- | --- | --- |
| MOSS | SALMON PINK | SALMON | RUST | LIGHT PEACH | PEACH |

# in your makeup bag

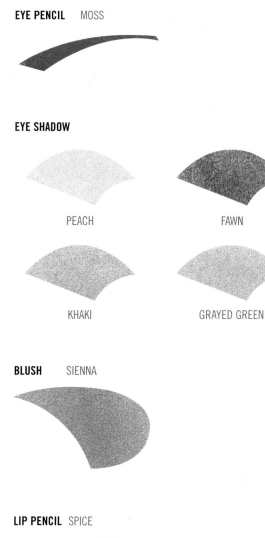

**EYE PENCIL**   MOSS

**EYE SHADOW**

PEACH

FAWN

KHAKI

GRAYED GREEN

**BLUSH**   SIENNA

**LIP PENCIL** SPICE

**LIPSTICK**   SANDALWOOD

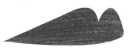

SPICED PEACH

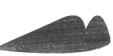

NUTMEG

# your face

- Your soft coloring needs to be complemented with makeup in soft, muted tones.
- For eye pencils try moss, brown, or coffee.
- Accent eye shadows such as khaki, grayed green, or brown will blend perfectly with peach, fawn, or toffee.
- Your blush will need to be soft and warm: try sienna.
- Soft lip pencils are best for you: use spice or natural.
- You will always need to wear lipstick to give you some definition. Balance your look with lipstick colors such as sandalwood, spiced peach, or nutmeg. Try lip gloss as an alternative: a natural, warm shade is good for you.

# your hair

- Your hair will be dark blonde or light to medium brown. If you highlight your hair, keep the colors warm and golden. A mix of hair colors will also work well for you: add rich, warm gold or copper tones to enhance the richness of the color.
- When natural gray highlights appear, just keep adding the highlights or lowlights as you have been doing. You can go golden, but if you change your hair color completely, your dominant coloring will change, too.

# mixing colors with confidence soft & warm

## warm-weather combinations

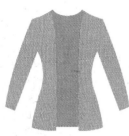

**BUSINESS WEAR**

sage + salmon
camel + natural beige
cocoa + peach
verbena + light moss

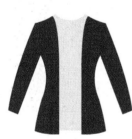

**CASUAL WEAR**

rust + shell
jade + light moss
taupe + golden brown
yellow-green + gray-green

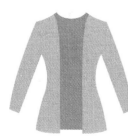

**SPECIAL OCCASION WEAR**

peach + salmon
salmon pink + rust
light moss + moss
light gold + buttermilk

## cool-weather combinations

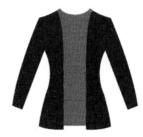

**BUSINESS WEAR**

chocolate + golden brown
teal + camel
moss + light moss
charcoal + salmon pink

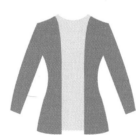

**CASUAL WEAR**

turquoise + yellow-green
spruce + rust
pewter + camel
cocoa + light gold

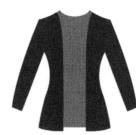

**SPECIAL OCCASION WEAR**

claret + salmon pink
jade + teal
damson + moss
rose brown + peach

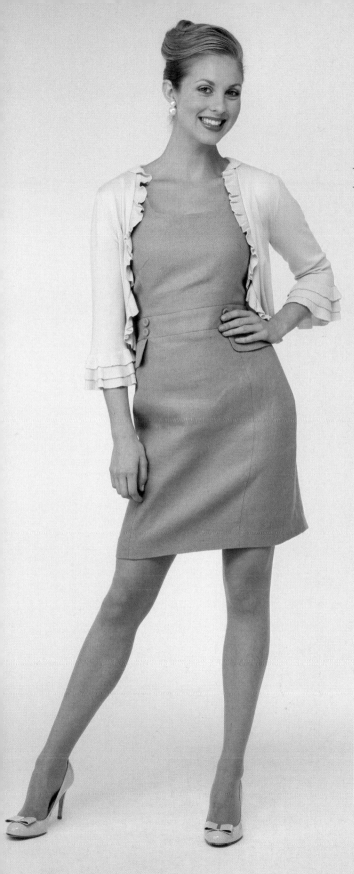

**LEFT** *Wearing your yellow green and light moss together, for a tone-on-tone look, is a fun way to wear colors.*

## ALTERNATIVE TO BLACK

The key to your look is to wear blended, not contrasting, shades. The tones of rose brown, pewter and cocoa in this outfit give an elegant look without overpowering the model's coloring. Light navy and charcoal gray are also great neutrals for a more formal look. When choosing your clothes, think about the fabric texture; tweeds, velours, and knits all help soften the color of many garments. Pearls and matte jewels are also a great choice for your coloring.

Now that you know your color palette, find out how to reflect your style through color: **go to pages 144–161**.

# soft & cool

- Take a close look at your hair color. Would you describe it as ash blonde or cool brown?
- Does your skin have a slightly pink tone? Do you tend to blush easily?
- Do you have smoky blue, green, or gray eyes?
- Do the color test with peach and orchid, and then with olive and sea green: *go to page 33*. You should find that your best pink is a cool shade such as orchid, and the cool tones of sea green will suit you better than warmer olive.

Your secondary characteristic is cool. Your additional colors will add coolness and depth to your main color palette.

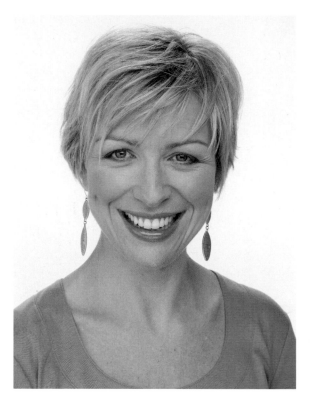

## your additional colors

As a Soft and Cool, you can now add these 12 extra shades to your master palette. When your are wearing warm colors like chocolate, rose brown, or verbena, mix them with cooler shades such as lavender, soft fuchsia or eau de nil for a more balanced look with your cool tones.

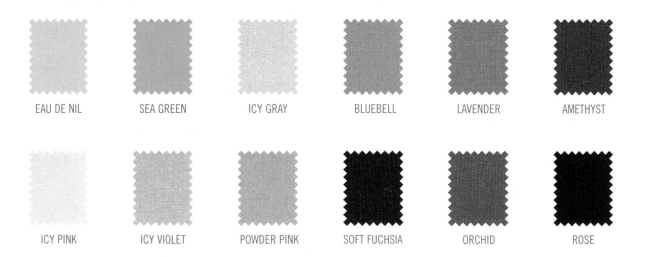

| EAU DE NIL | SEA GREEN | ICY GRAY | BLUEBELL | LAVENDER | AMETHYST |
| --- | --- | --- | --- | --- | --- |
| ICY PINK | ICY VIOLET | POWDER PINK | SOFT FUCHSIA | ORCHID | ROSE |

# in your makeup bag

**EYE PENCIL**    COFFEE

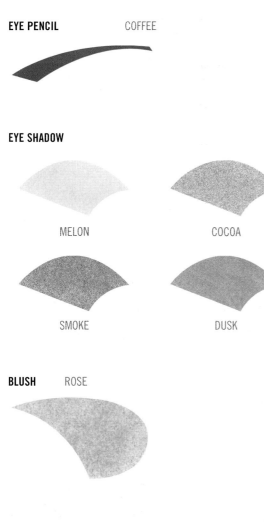

**EYE SHADOW**

MELON

COCOA

SMOKE

DUSK

**BLUSH**    ROSE

**LIP PENCIL**  NATURAL

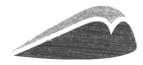

**LIPSTICK**  MULBERRY

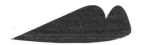

SOFT MAUVE

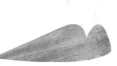

PINK SHELL

# your face

- Your soft coloring needs to be complemented with cool, muted makeup shades; avoid using color combinations that are too contrasting.
- For eye pencils try coffee, eggplant, granite, or dark blue.
- Accent eye shadows such as cocoa, heather, or smoky blues and grays work well with melon, dusk, and pale pinks.
- Your blush will need to be soft and cool: try rose or candy pink.
- Cool shades of lip pencil work best, so try natural or pink.
- Balance your whole look with soft, cool lipsticks like mulberry, soft mauve, or dusty rose. Lip gloss also works well for you: try pink shell.

# your hair

- You will have dark blonde to light or medium brown hair that has ash, rather than honey-colored, undertones to it.
- You will probably already be highlighting your hair; keep to cool platinum or ash shades and avoid red or coppery tones.
- When natural gray highlights appear, just keep adding the highlights or lowlights as you have been.

# mixing colors with confidence soft & cool

## warm-weather combinations

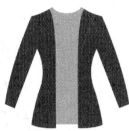

**BUSINESS WEAR**
charcoal blue + bluebell
jade + sea green
taupe + icy gray
light periwinkle + lavender

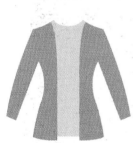

**CASUAL WEAR**
sky blue + eau de nil
blush pink + rose
shell + rose brown
emerald turquoise + turquoise

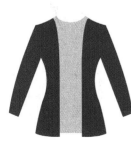

**SPECIAL OCCASION WEAR**
rose + powder pink
light periwinkle + icy gray
sage + gray-green
soft violet + icy violet

## cool-weather combinations

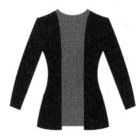

**BUSINESS WEAR**
light navy + orchid
charcoal + amethyst
teal + jade
rose brown + powder pink

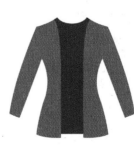

**CASUAL WEAR**
blush pink + rose
damson + amethyst
spruce + sage
charcoal + soft fuchsia

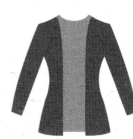

**SPECIAL OCCASION WEAR**
amethyst + lavender
sapphire + bluebell
claret + orchid
emerald turquoise + sea green

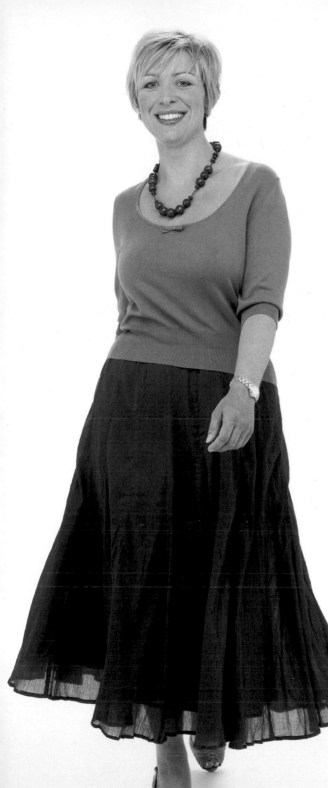

**LEFT** *Light periwinkle and amethyst are a perfect combination for someone who is Soft and Cool.*

## ALTERNATIVE TO BLACK

The blended tones of gray in this dress give a wonderful Soft and Cool look. Other alternatives for you to try are teal, charcoal blue, light navy, and spruce. Use tonal colors with these neutrals to avoid high contrast. It is much more flattering to wear tone-on-tone shades from the same color palette. Your makeup should be Soft and Cool and tone in with the colors you are wearing.

Now that you know your color palette, find out how to reflect your style through color: **go to pages 144–161.**

# how to wear black

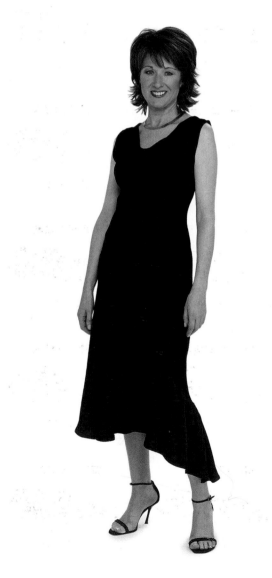

It is commonly believed that black is slimming. This is, however, only true if it is worn in the correct style and fabric. As we have seen earlier in this chapter, there are many alternatives to black in everyone's palette to make them look appropriate for work or formal occasions, and slimmer, too. At **colour me beautiful** we believe that it is not the color you wear but how you wear it that makes it a success. Over the following pages we will demonstrate that, whatever your coloring, black can be worn successfully even if it doesn't appear in your palette.

## the key to success

Everyone can still have their LBD depending on the fabric, how much skin is on show, and what accessories and makeup are worn.

### ALL SHADES OF BLACK

Texture and weave will affect the way in which light is absorbed by the fabric. The appearance of black will soften when you use a textured fabric; this is a great way for Softs and Lights to introduce black into their wardrobe. All types of knits, both synthetic and pure wool, will soften black, as well as tweeds. Sheer fabrics also "lighten" black, and shiny fabrics, such as silk or satin, will sparkle and reflect the light.

## SHOWING SKIN

Very few women—except the Deeps—will be able to wear a black turtleneck sweater. Indeed, a Deep is the only coloring type that can wear a dark color on its own near the face. To help wear black successfully, leave enough skin on show with a lower or open neckline.

## ACCESSORIZE YOUR BLACK WITH SCARVES

Scarves are a wonderful addition to any wardrobe and are a foolproof ally to ensure that black works for you, whatever your coloring. Choose your scarf in your favorite color(s) and wear it near your face so that the colors reflecting onto your face are in harmony and balance with your natural coloring. There are many ways of wearing scarves, and they will add style depending on what shape they are (pashmina style, large square, oblong) and how you wear them.

## ACCESSORIZE YOUR BLACK WITH JEWELRY

Wearing jewelry, whether real or costume, is a surefire way to make your black outfit flattering. The light will reflect on metals and beads, giving a lift and bringing out your natural coloring. Make sure that the color of the beads are in your palette. Warmer skin tones are best in gold, copper, and bronze; cooler skin tones are best in silver, platinum, and pewter. Diamonds are perfect on everyone!

## MAKEUP

Make sure that you are wearing the right shades of makeup for your color palette: *go to pages 34–105*. Many women make the mistake of wearing too strong a shade of lipstick or blush when wearing black, especially in the evening. Also avoid the temptation to be overdramatic with your eyeliner and eye shadow colors.

# wearing lipstick with black

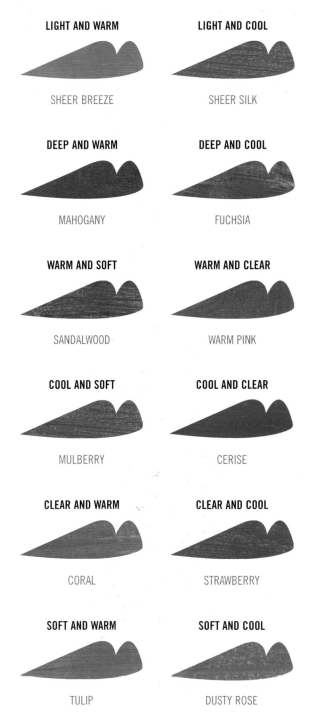

**LIGHT AND WARM**
SHEER BREEZE

**LIGHT AND COOL**
SHEER SILK

**DEEP AND WARM**
MAHOGANY

**DEEP AND COOL**
FUCHSIA

**WARM AND SOFT**
SANDALWOOD

**WARM AND CLEAR**
WARM PINK

**COOL AND SOFT**
MULBERRY

**COOL AND CLEAR**
CERISE

**CLEAR AND WARM**
CORAL

**CLEAR AND COOL**
STRAWBERRY

**SOFT AND WARM**
TULIP

**SOFT AND COOL**
DUSTY ROSE

| LIGHT | DEEP | WARM |
|---|---|---|

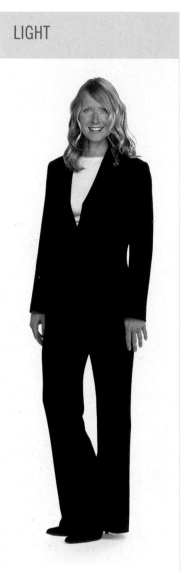

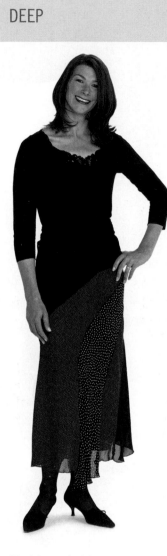

Team your black business suit with one of your light shades, such as dusty rose, yellow green, or primrose. Avoid the temptation to wear it with white. For evening, try a black lacy or chiffon top.

Black is wonderful on you, because it balances your deep, rich coloring. Wear it as much as you want on its own or with other colors from your palette.

Black is not in your palette, but make sure that you have one of your best colors, such as coral pink or salmon, near your face.

## COOL

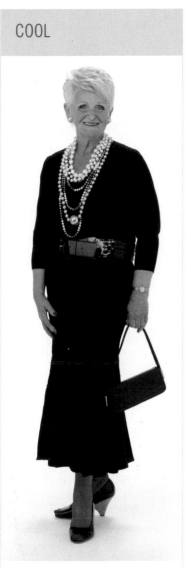

Black is a key color in your palette, but it needs to be contrasted with a lighter or brighter color; alternatively, pile on the jewelry to create a light-reflecting effect around your neck and face.

## CLEAR

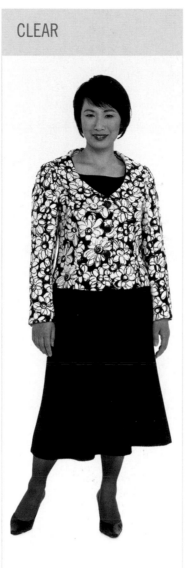

Black and pure white is a stunning combination for day and night, for any occasion. You can also combine black with any pale or striking colors from your palette.

## SOFT

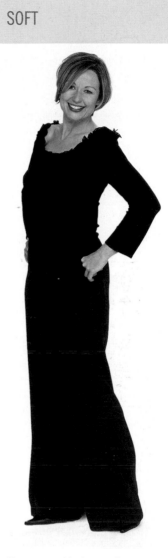

Always wear black away from your face, and choose fabrics that are textured or soft to the touch, such as knits. Details such as frills, velvet, or chiffon trims will all help soften the look.

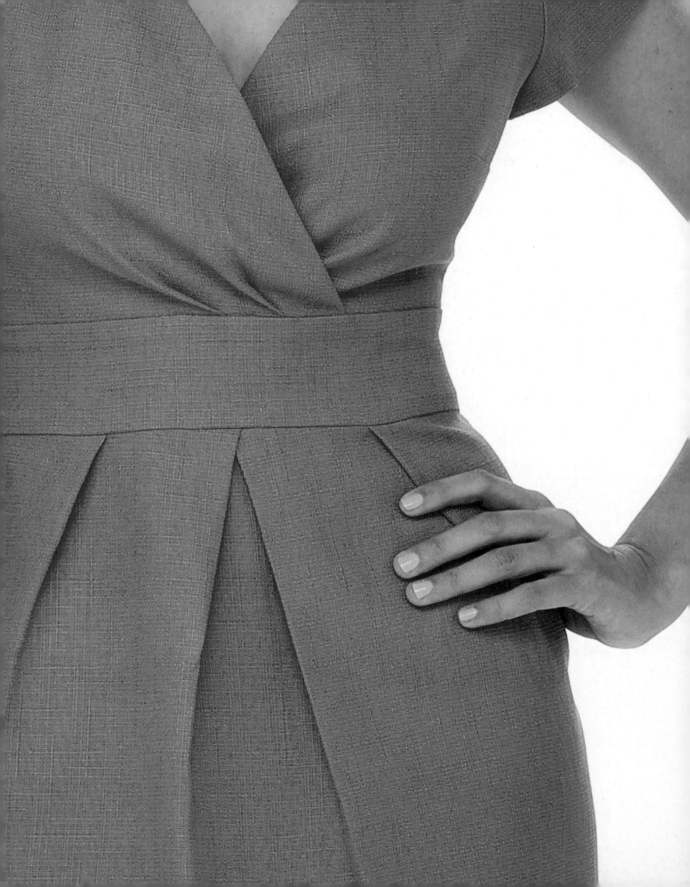

# 3

# size doesn't matter, shape does

# women should have curves

WHILE FASHION MAGAZINES MAY BE FULL OF WAIFLIKE MODELS WITH FRAGILE, STICK-THIN LIMBS AND BODIES AS FLAT AS BOARDS, WOMEN ARE ACTUALLY DESIGNED TO HAVE CURVES. IT'S NATURAL, IT'S FEMININE, IT'S SEXY—AND MOST MEN SAY THEY PREFER CURVY WOMEN.

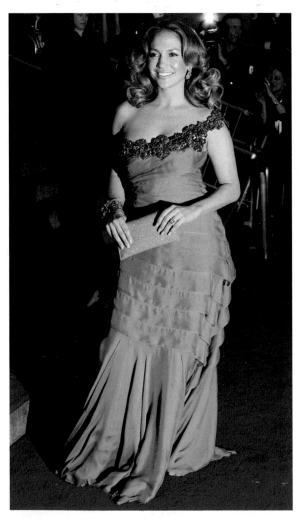

*Jennifer Lopez is widely admired for her fantastic hourglass curves and shapely derrière.*

When it comes to looking good, it's not your size or shape that matters, it's the fit of your clothes. Wearing the right clothes is not about following the latest fashion or fad, it's about choosing what actually suits you—not your best friend—and what makes you feel comfortable and confident.

By knowing your basic body shape and understanding the guidelines for choosing the types of clothes that will accentuate your good features and minimize your less-than-perfect areas, you will be able to dress in the way that suits you best. You will also be able to see how to make subtle changes to the way you put your wardrobe together.

Today, the choice of clothes is so varied that you should always be able to find something that will complement your body shape, scale, proportions, and coloring.

## body shapes

Clothing is either constructed along straight lines, which give a garment a more rigid, structured form, or along curved lines, which give a more fluid shape that tends to follow the curves of the body.

You cannot change your basic body line by diet or exercise. It will remain essentially the same throughout your life, because your body line is based on your skeleton as well as your genes. The distribution of body fat is also dependent on your genes. If you have a tendency to carry extra weight on your hips, you will almost certainly have a proportionally smaller waist; conversely, women who carry extra weight around their tummies will have straight hips and bottoms.

Biologically, women are designed to carry more fat beneath their skin than men (the original hunter-gatherers), and we actually need a few curves in order for our bodies to work efficiently. Fatty deposits around the hips, legs, and arms are normal and should not be viewed as worrying health indicators (unless you are grossly overweight).

When most women stand in front of a mirror, they focus on all the things they would like to change about their bodies. On the following pages you will learn how to recognize your assets and show them off, and how to play down the parts of your body that you are not so happy with. The objective is for you to understand your shape, to be positive about it, and to make the most of what nature has given you.

Whether you are petite or have a fuller figure, the cut of the clothes that will flatter you best will depend on your basic body shape. For example, if you have a Full Hourglass figure, wearing softer lines is recommended. The only difference between what suits a petite or fuller-figured woman of this body shape will be the size of the pattern and the weight of the fabric in which the garment is made.

## the illusion of a balanced body

When choosing clothes, your aim is to create the illusion of having a balanced body: a Neat Hourglass figure with:

• Shoulders and hips in line
• A defined bust
• A waist, even with a softly curved tummy
• A curved bottom
• Perfect proportions

# what body shape are you?

TO IDENTIFY YOUR BASIC BODY SHAPE, ANSWER THE QUESTIONS IN THE BOXES BELOW. IF YOU DON'T FIT EXACTLY INTO JUST ONE SHAPE, CHOOSE THE ONE THAT MOST CLOSELY RESEMBLES YOU. THEN TURN TO THE RELEVANT SECTION TO DISCOVER YOUR CLOTHING GUIDELINES.

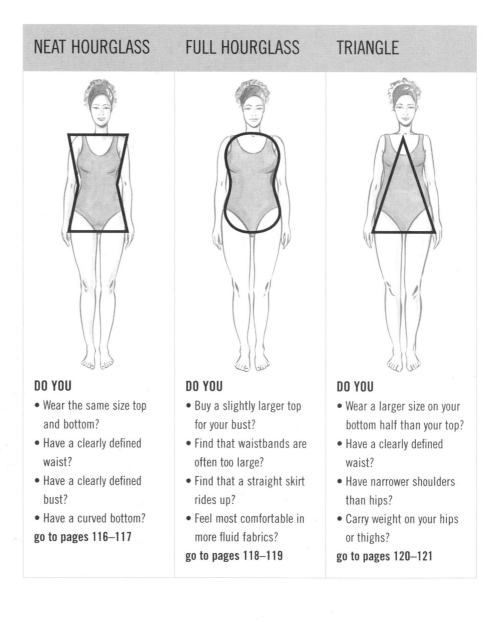

| NEAT HOURGLASS | FULL HOURGLASS | TRIANGLE |
|---|---|---|

**DO YOU**
- Wear the same size top and bottom?
- Have a clearly defined waist?
- Have a clearly defined bust?
- Have a curved bottom?

**go to pages 116–117**

**DO YOU**
- Buy a slightly larger top for your bust?
- Find that waistbands are often too large?
- Find that a straight skirt rides up?
- Feel most comfortable in more fluid fabrics?

**go to pages 118–119**

**DO YOU**
- Wear a larger size on your bottom half than your top?
- Have a clearly defined waist?
- Have narrower shoulders than hips?
- Carry weight on your hips or thighs?

**go to pages 120–121**

| INVERTED TRIANGLE | LEAN COLUMN | RECTANGLE | ROUND |
|---|---|---|---|

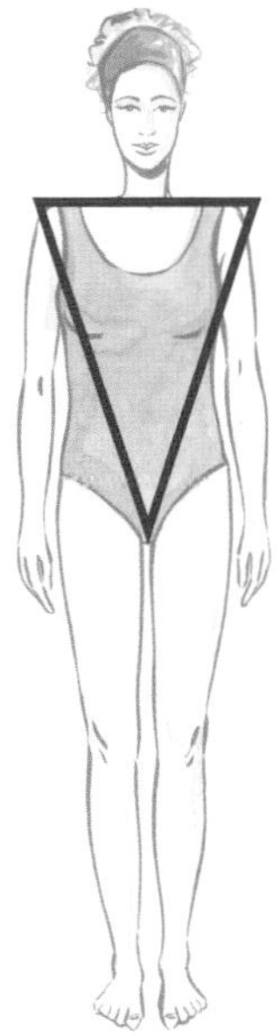

**DO YOU**

- Wear a larger size on your top half than your bottom?
- Have wider shoulders than hips?
- Have a straight rib cage?
- Prefer an uncluttered look?

**go to pages 122–123**

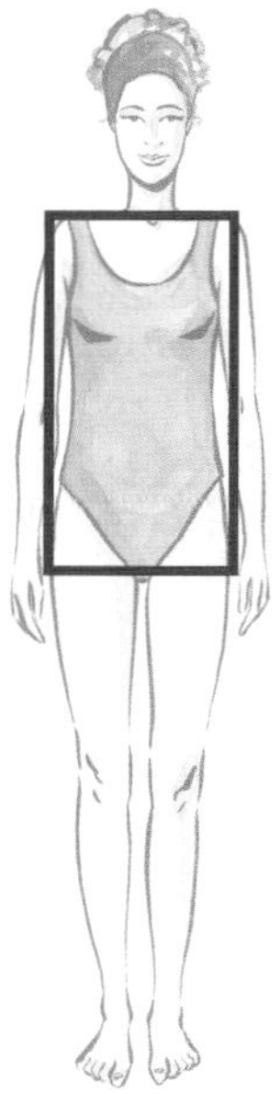

**DO YOU**

- Wear the same size on your top and bottom halves?
- Have a minimal bust?
- Have little waist definition?
- Have flat hips and bottom?

**go to pages 124–125**

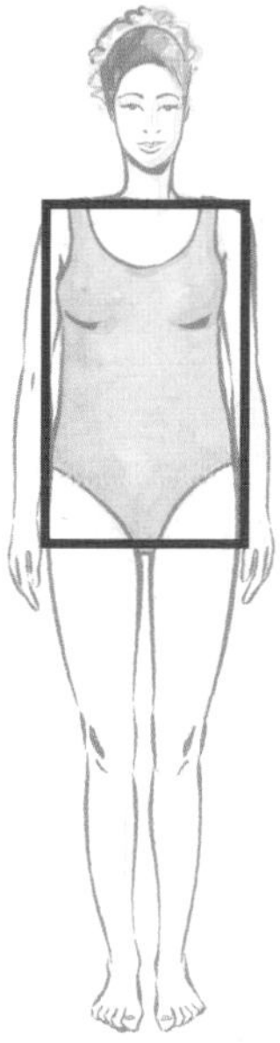

**DO YOU**

- Have shoulders and hips in line?
- Have no waist definition?
- Have flat hips and bottom?
- Carry any extra weight around your middle?

**go to pages 126–127**

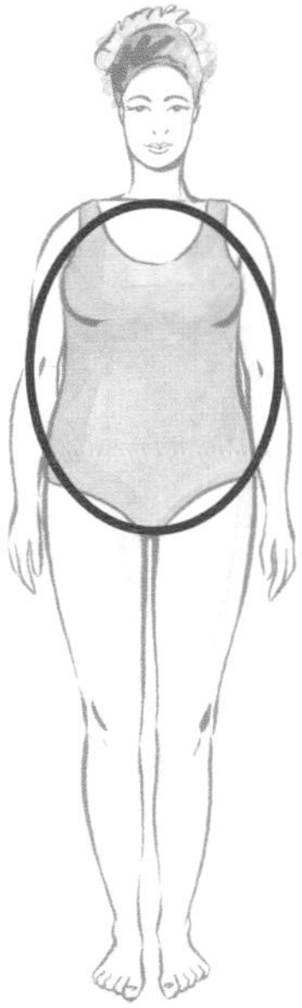

**DO YOU**

- Have rounded shoulders?
- Have fullness in the tummy area?
- Have wonderfully shapely legs?
- Feel uncomfortable when clothes are tucked in?

**go to pages 128–129**

# neat hourglass

LUCKY YOU! YOU HAVE A BALANCED BODY WITH YOUR TOP HALF IN PROPORTION TO YOUR BOTTOM HALF. THIS MEANS THAT YOUR CLOTHES DON'T NEED TO WORK HARD AT EVENING OUT YOUR SHAPE AND CAN SIMPLY FOLLOW YOUR NATURAL CURVES.

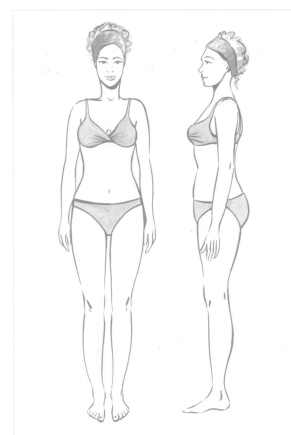

## YOUR BUILD IS CHARACTERIZED BY

- A defined bust
- A defined waist
- A neat bottom
- Neat hips

## your golden rules

- Show off your body by wearing clothes that define your waist, enhance your bust, and highlight your hips and bottom.
- Avoid wearing clothes that hide your body line, or you risk looking an extra seven to nine pounds (three to four kilos) heavier than you are.

## your clothing lines

**Jackets** Fitted, with waist definition.

**Tops** Shaped, crossovers, or wraps.

**Skirts** Straight, paneled, flip, bias cut, soft pleats or full, preferably with a waistband and some shaping (darts) over the hips and bottom.

**Pants** Any type, with a waistband (see above).

**Jeans** Designed for women's bodies.

**Dresses** Any style, either shaped or belted.

**Coats** All shapes, as long as they have a belt or some shape at the waist.

**Swimwear** As long as your proportions are good, you can wear any style (see illustration left).

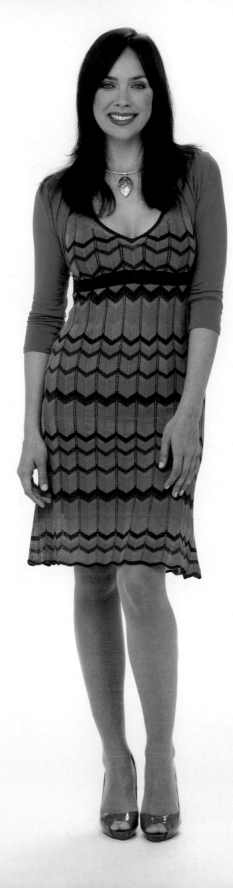

## your best fabrics

Choose fabrics that are light to medium in weight and texture. These will skim the curves of your body:

Cotton

Linen

Silk

Tightly woven gabardine to relaxed wool crepe

All jerseys and polyesters

All knits

## your best patterns

Because the top and bottom half of your body are in balance, you are able to wear most types of pattern.

Stripes

Abstract

Checks

Polka dots

Florals

Paisleys

## you should avoid

Boxy jackets

Pants or skirts that have no shaping

Straight tunics

Men's shirts

Baggy sweaters and sportswear

Too much layering

For more on proportions and scale: **go to pages 136–138**; for more on who can wear what: **go to pages 130–135**.

# full hourglass

LUCKY YOU! YOU HAVE THE MOST FEMININE BODY SHAPE, WITH FULL CURVES IN ALL THE RIGHT PLACES. BY CHOOSING CLOTHES THAT ARE FLUID AND SHAPED, YOU WILL BE ABLE TO ACCENTUATE YOUR CURVES RATHER THAN COVER THEM UP.

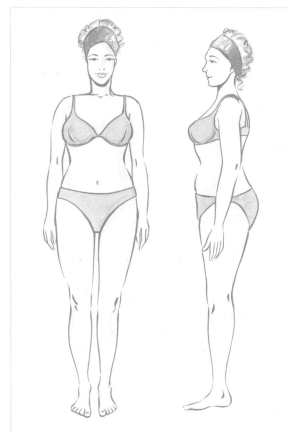

## YOUR BUILD IS CHARACTERIZED BY
- A full bust
- A small waist
- A rounded bottom
- Rounded hips

## your golden rules
- It is important that you wear clothes that follow your body line as opposed to those that are straight and constrict you.
- Choose fabrics carefully. Avoid heavy or stiff materials, or you'll end up with tops and jackets that are two to three sizes bigger than you need just to accommodate your curves.

## your clothing lines
**Jackets** Shaped, with shawl collars or concealed front openings.
**Tops** Shaped, crossovers, or wraps, in soft fabrics.
**Skirts** Flip, bias or full, and adjustable at the waist.
**Pants** Flat-fronted with side zipper.
**Dresses** Shaped, wrap, or bias-cut sheath.
**Coats** Shawl collar, single-breasted, or shaped.
**Swimwear** Underwiring or support is essential. Avoid stripes and detailing at the bust and hips (see illustration left).

## your best fabrics

Should be light to medium weight, with little texture. If choosing cotton or linen, look for fabrics cut on the bias to give movement and accommodate your curves:

Silk and chiffon

Relaxed wool crepe

All jerseys and polyesters

Fine knits

Fabric that gives and stretches

Lycra, the best friend of the Full Hourglass

## your best patterns

Avoid geometric patterns, because lines will not lie straight over your curves. Instead, opt for more fluid shapes such as:

Polka dots

Florals

Paisleys

Circles and squiggles

## you should avoid

Jeans (too many pockets)

Straight skirts, except in soft fabrics with some Lycra

Boxy, double-breasted jackets

Straight tunics

Front-opening shirts and blouses

Baggy sweaters and sportswear

Too much layering

Crisp fabrics

Stripes and checks

For more on proportions and scale: **go to pages 136–138**; for more on who can wear what: **go to pages 130–135**.

# triangle

LUCKY YOU! YOU CAN BRING ALL THE ATTENTION TO THE TOP HALF OF YOUR BODY. YOU ARE OFTEN REFERRED TO AS PEAR-SHAPED, SO WITH YOUR CHOICE OF CLOTHES YOU SHOULD AIM TO ACCENTUATE YOUR BUST AND MINIMIZE YOUR BOTTOM AND HIPS.

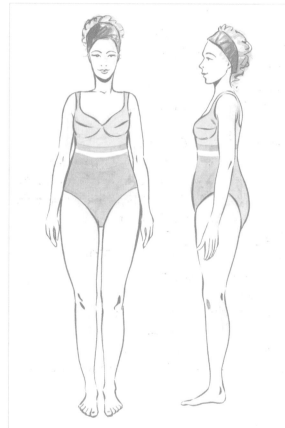

## YOUR BUILD IS CHARACTERIZED BY

- Full hips or thighs
- A defined waist
- Shoulders that may slope and are narrower than your hips
- A top half that appears small

## your golden rules

- Your jackets and tops need to finish either above or below the widest point of your hips and bottom.
- Layering on your top half creates visual interest and draws the eye upward.
- Buy jackets or tops that fit your shoulders rather than your hips—you can always leave the bottom button undone.

## your clothing lines

**Jackets** Details, collars, pockets, buttons, or double-breasted are excellent.

**Tops** Patterned, horizontal stripes, or twinsets.

**Skirts** Simple lines: long flip, bias cut, or paneled.

**Pants** Plain, flat-fronted with side zipper, bootleg, or flared (for long legs).

**Dresses** Separates work better.

**Coats** Square shoulders or wide collars.

**Swimwear** Keep detailing above the waist. Beware of high-cut styles that finish at your widest point (see illustration left).

## your best fabrics

Your aim is to balance out your body shape, so certain fabrics will work best on your lower half: Light- to medium-weight fabrics with minimum texture are best.
Soft, fluid fabrics that drape easily, such as wool crepe, jersey, knits, fabrics cut on the bias, silks.

Other fabrics that will flatter and draw attention to your top half are:
Light fabrics worn layered
Medium- to heavyweight fabrics
Texture, which adds volume
Cotton and linen
All types of woolen fabrics
Crisper fabrics, which add bulk

## your best patterns

Any pattern, such as florals or horizontal stripes, is a great way to draw attention to the upper half of your body. Always wear plain colors below the waist.

## you should avoid

Jeans (too many pockets)
Straight skirts
Details on skirts and pants
Halter necks and raglan sleeves
Tight-fitting, single-layered tops
Tops and jackets that finish at your widest point

For more on proportions and scale: **go to pages 136–138**; for more on who can wear what: **go to pages 130–135**.

# inverted triangle

LUCKY YOU! YOU HAVE GREAT SHOULDERS—HALTER NECKS ARE MADE FOR YOU. TO BALANCE THE UPPER AND LOWER PARTS OF YOUR BODY, YOU NEED TO HIGHLIGHT YOUR HIPS AND BOTTOM, FOCUSING ALL ATTENTION BELOW YOUR WAIST.

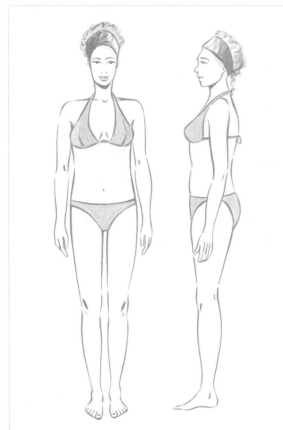

## YOUR BUILD IS CHARACTERIZED BY
- Straight and squared shoulder line
- Little definition between waist/hips
- Flat hips and bottom
- A bottom half that seems smaller than your top half

## your golden rules
- You will need to keep detail to a minimum on your shoulder line; keep this area as simple as possible.
- Your clothing lines need to be straight, clean, and sharp.
- Your silhouette should be uncluttered.

## your clothing lines

**Jackets** Constructed, or shaped with angular lines (collars with lapels).

**Tops** Simple lines.

**Skirts** Straight, box pleats or paneled.

**Pants** Any style—pockets and details will accentuate your bottom.

**Dresses** Simple, straight lines or sheaths.

**Coats** Straight lines with a slightly shaped waistline and no belt.

**Swimwear** Halter and square necklines work well, as do details on the hips (see illustration left). Avoid floral patterns. Go for styles where tops and bottoms are sold separately.

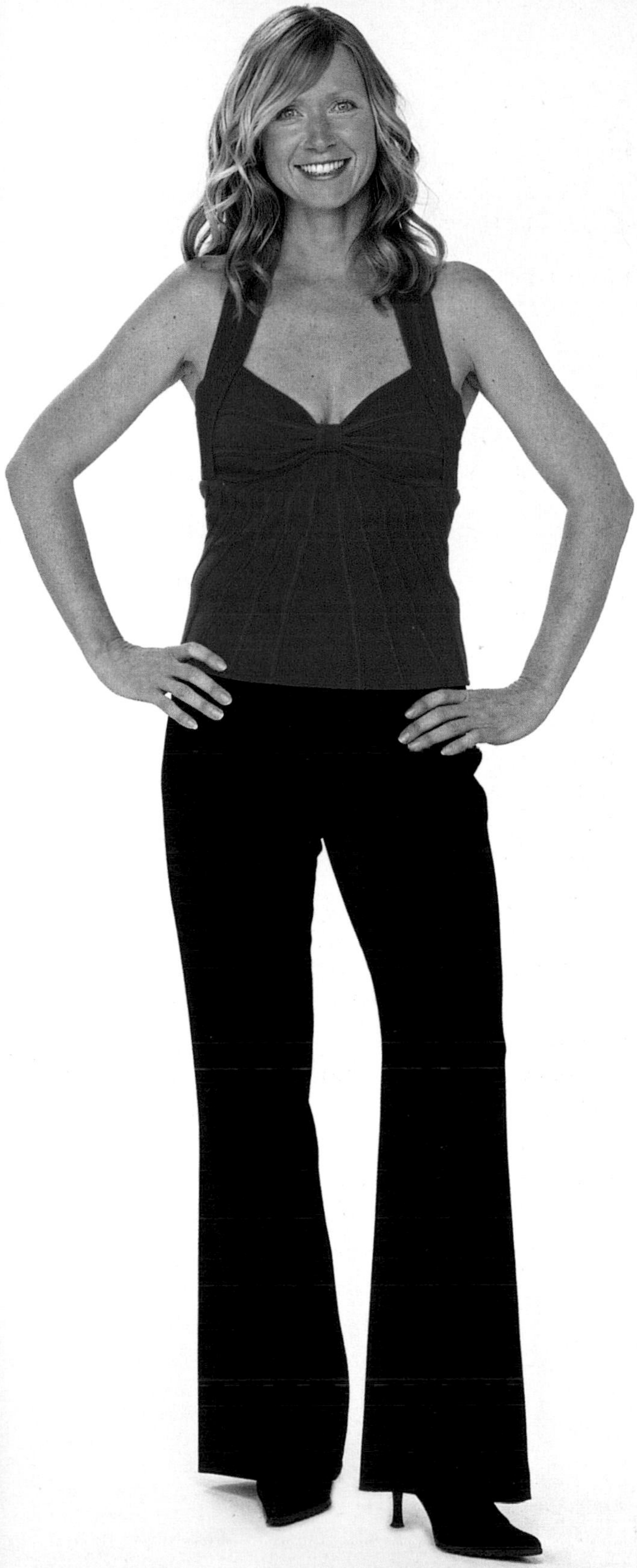

## your best fabrics

Crisp, constructed fabrics work best for you because your body line is straight and angled.

Crisp cottons and linens
Gabardine and fine wool
Satins and crisp silks
Crinkled fabrics

## your best patterns

You can wear patterns above and below the waistline, but they must be geometric to balance the clothing line.

Stripes
Checks
Geometrics
Squiggles and dots

## you should avoid

Frills and flounces
Gathered waistlines
Tiered skirts
Epaulettes
Soft, floppy, and fluffy fabrics
Bias cuts

For more on proportions and scale: **go to pages 136–138**; for more on who can wear what: **go to pages 130–135**.

# lean column

LUCKY YOU! YOU'VE GOT THE FIGURE OF A RUNWAY MODEL. YOUR CHALLENGE IS TO CREATE AN ILLUSION OF CURVES WHERE THERE ARE NONE, SO GO FOR DESIGNS WITH SHAPE AND DETAIL THAT EMPHASIZE YOUR BUST, HIPS, AND BOTTOM AND DEFINE YOUR WAIST.

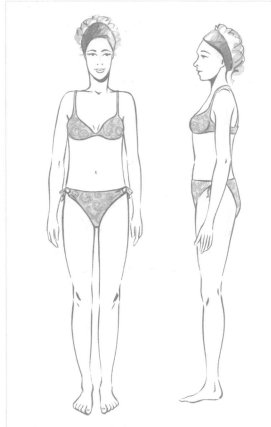

## YOUR BUILD IS CHARACTERIZED BY
- Narrow shoulders and lean limbs
- Flat chest or small bust
- Small and non-defined waist
- Narrow hips and flat bottom

## your golden rules
- Highlight your hips and bottom.
- Enhance your bustline with details.
- Your clothing line needs to be straight, with emphasis on the waist.
- Use texture and layering.

## your clothing lines
**Jackets** Waisted jackets, with details or pockets.
**Tops** Details, textures, patterns, and layers.
**Skirts** A-line, paneled, gored, or pleated.
**Pants** Shaped, pleated, and pocketed.
**Dresses** Princess line with curved darts and details on the bust and hips.
**Coats** Martingale, shaped.
**Swimwear** Padded styles are perfect. Use patterned two-pieces to emphasize your bust and hips (see illustration left). Vertical chevron lines on a one-piece will give the illusion of shape.

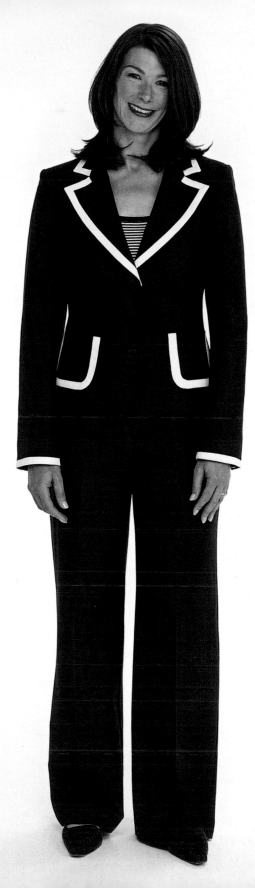

## your best fabrics

Textured fabrics or fabrics that you can layer are both good choices for you.

Cottons and linens

Gabardine, fine wool, and lightweight tweeds

Satins and silks

Crinkled fabrics

Light, woven textures

## your best patterns

Wearing pattern on your top half will draw the eye and emphasize your bust, while clothing details such as pockets will accentuate your hips.

Squiggles, paisleys, and dots

Horizontal stripes

Checks

Geometrics

Discreet florals

## you should avoid

Full frills and flounces

Large, gathered skirts

Belted jackets and coats

Bulky, heavy textures

Close-fitting, figure-hugging garments

For more on proportions and scale: **go to pages 136–138**; for more on who can wear what: **go to pages 130–135.**

# rectangle

LUCKY YOU! YOU ARE THE ONE WITH FLAT HIPS AND A FLAT BOTTOM. HOWEVER, SOME RECTANGLES WILL HAVE A FULLER BUST, GIVING A SOFTER EDGE TO THEIR SHAPE. YOUR MAIN AIM IS TO SOFTEN THOSE EDGES EVEN MORE AND CREATE THE APPEARANCE OF CURVES.

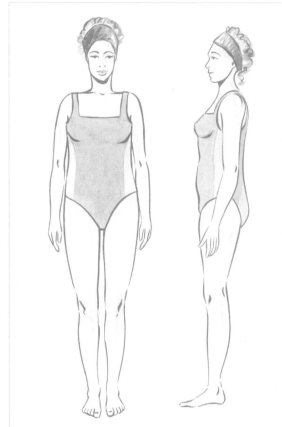

## YOUR BUILD IS CHARACTERIZED BY

- Straight shoulder line
- Straight hips and bottom
- Very little waist definition
- Straight ribcage

## your golden rules

- Use details on your hips and bottom to create shape.
- Avoid details at the waist, such as noticeable waistbands or belts.
- Keep your clothing lines straight.
- Go for the uncluttered look.

## your clothing lines

**Jackets** Structured and shaped.
**Tops** Simple, clean lines.
**Skirts** Crossover, straight, box pleats, or paneled.
**Pants** The choice is yours.
**Dresses** Simple, straight lines or sheaths.
**Coats** Straight lines with some emphasis on the waist.
**Swimwear** On a one-piece, a central panel in a darker shade gives the illusion of a slimmer shape, as do square necklines (see illustration left). Avoid high-waisted bikini bottoms, and choose geometric patterns.

## your best fabrics

Most Rectangles can wear crisp fabrics, but if you have a full bust, slightly softer fabrics work better.
Wool crepe and woven wool
Cottons and linens
Jersey and lightweight tweeds
Fine knits

## your best patterns

Geometric patterns work best for you because your body is straight.
Vertical stripes
Checks
Geometrics
Squiggles and dots

## you should avoid

Frills and flounces
Gathered waistlines
Soft, floppy, and fluffy fabrics
Bias cuts
Belted jackets and coats
Florals and paisleys

For more on proportions and scale: **go to pages 136–138**; for more on who can wear what: **go to pages 130–135**.

# round

LUCKY YOU! YOU'VE GOT GREAT LEGS. YOUR PROBLEM AREA IS YOUR CENTRAL TORSO, SO WHEREVER POSSIBLE USE ACCESSORIES TO DRAW THE EYE TO THE AREA ABOVE YOUR BUST AND BELOW YOUR HIPS. YOUR AIM IS TO GIVE THE IMPRESSION OF A SLIGHTLY LONGER BODY.

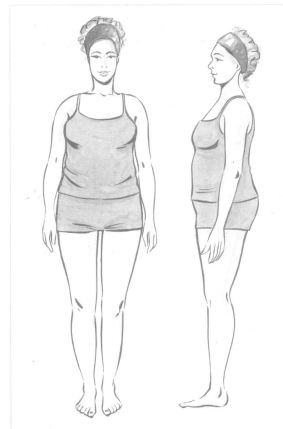

## YOUR BUILD IS CHARACTERIZED BY
- Rounded shoulder line
- Curved back
- Fullness around the middle
- Flattish bottom

## your golden rules
- Make sure the clothes you wear hang from your shoulders.
- Clothing lines need to be straight, and fabrics soft, to avoid any unnecessary volume or bulkiness.
- Keep any detail above the bustline and below the hipline.
- Accessorize, accessorize, accessorize.

## your clothing lines
**Jackets** Cardigan-style, collarless, shawl collar, V-shaped neckline.
**Tops** Simple lines, no details.
**Skirts** Wrap, flip, or paneled.
**Pants** Drawstrings, no waistband.
**Dresses** A-line (trapeze).
**Coats** A-line, cardigan-style.
**Swimwear** Try a tankini or tank top that covers the middle and isn't too figure-hugging (see illustration left). For more cover, use a sarong. Details on the shoulders draw the eye toward your face.

## your best fabrics

The key is to choose soft, fluid fabrics that hang well and don't cling or hug the figure. Stiff or thick fabric will add unwelcome girth.

Soft cottons and linens
Wool crepe
Jersey
Knits
Silks

## your best patterns

Try to go for muted and subtle patterns as much as possible; anything too bold will overpower.

Soft or faded stripes
Squiggles and dots
Abstract florals or paisleys

## you should avoid

Stiff fabrics
Pockets
Gathered waistlines or any other details over the tummy area
Sharp, angular details such as lapels
Vibrant and dramatic patterns over the torso

For more on proportions and scale: **go to pages 136–138**; for more on who can wear what: **go to pages 130–135**.

# who can wear what

BY RECOGNIZING THE SUBTLE DIFFERENCES IN THE STYLING OF CLOTHES, YOU WILL BE ABLE TO CHOOSE EXACTLY THE RIGHT TYPE OF JACKET, SKIRT, TOP, AND SO ON TO FLATTER YOUR BODY SHAPE AND SO ENHANCE YOUR OVERALL LOOK.

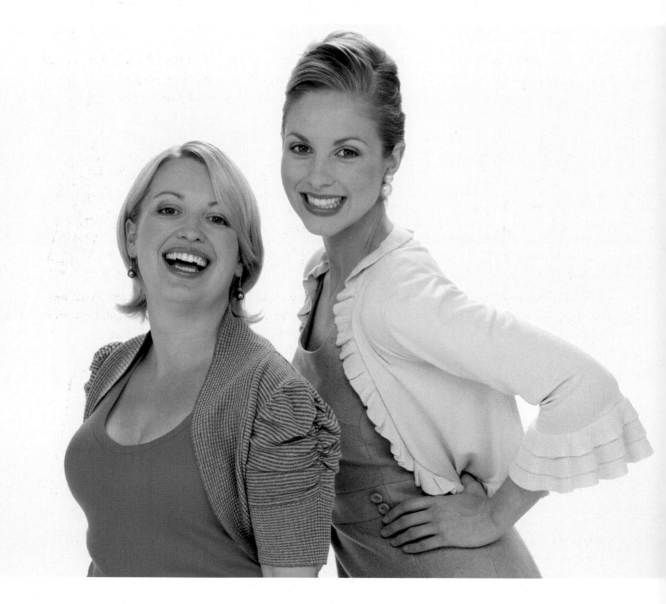

# jackets

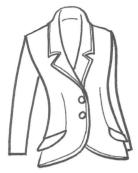

**Fitted with waist definition**
Good for emphasizing and
enhancing waistlines.

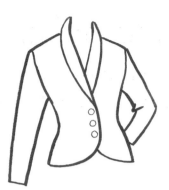

**Shaped with shawl collar** The
best shape for Full Hourglasses.
Make sure the jacket closes.

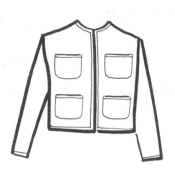

**Detailed** Adds interest to bust
and hips, so good for Lean
Columns and Rectangles.

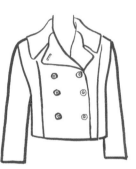

**Double-breasted** Great for
Triangles, but not in long-lined
blazer styles.

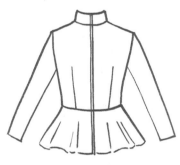

**Fitted with peplum** Good
for Neat Hourglasses, Lean
Columns, and Rectangles.

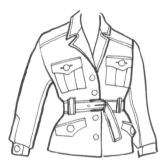

**Safari** Neat Hourglasses and
Lean Columns will look great
in this style jacket.

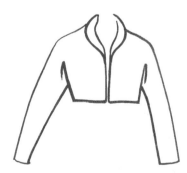

**Cropped** A great look for
adding volume to the top half
for Triangles.

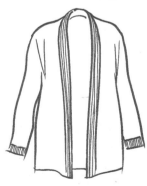

**Cardigan style** A relaxed
style perfect for Rounds and
Full Hourglasses.

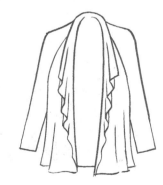

**Waterfall** A soft style that
will fall gently over anyone
with a full bust.

# tops

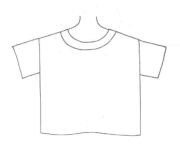

**Wide t-shape** Perfect for Rounds or women with a very full bust.

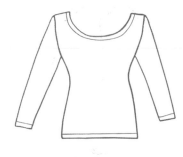

**Shaped** Good for most body shapes, except round.

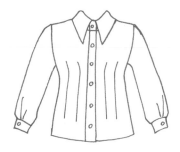

**Fitted shirt** Great on Neat Hourglasses, Inverted Triangles, and Lean Columns.

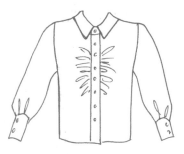

**Gathered** This is the shirt to wear in soft fabrics to enhance the bust.

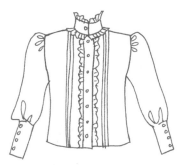

**Detailed blouse** Good for those with small busts, Triangles, and Lean Columns.

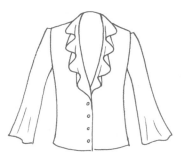

**Ruffle** Good on fuller busts as long as the fabric is soft and falls flat.

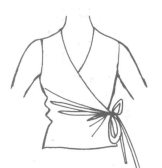

**Crossover/wrap** Can be worn layered, so good for Triangles; tied at the back.

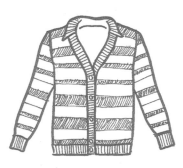

**Stripes or patterned** Good for Lean Columns and those wishing to enhance their bust.

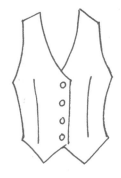

**Vest** Will add volume to the top half of Triangles and are good for Lean Columns.

# skirts

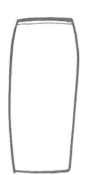

**Straight** Good for Inverted Triangles, Rectangles, and Neat Hourglasses.

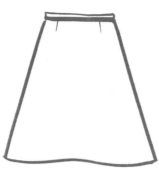

**A-line** These skirts give width to the hips, so are perfect for Inverted Triangles.

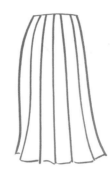

**Paneled** Works on all body shapes; if you have curvy hips, choose soft fabrics.

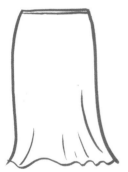

**Flip** Long or short, this skirt is flattering and great fun to wear for all body shapes.

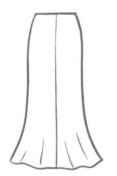

**Bias cut** This is perfect for Neat and Full Hourglasses and also Triangles.

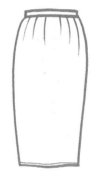

**Shaped** Ideal for those who have a well-defined waist, so good for Hourglasses.

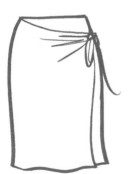

**Crossover/wrap** Good on all body shapes where the waistline might need adjustment.

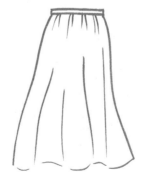

**Soft pleats** These will hang perfectly over the hips of Neat and Full Hourglasses.

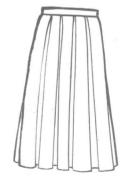

**Box pleats** Great for Inverted Triangles and Rectangles with flat hips.

# pants

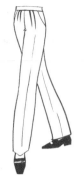

**Classic pleated with waistband** Perfect for Neat Hourglasses and Triangles.

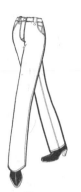

**Classic jeans** Best worn by Inverted Triangles, Lean Columns, and Rectangles.

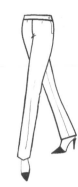

**Narrow** These will give the illusion of longer legs, but best avoided by Triangles.

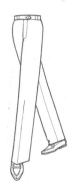

**Straight** Works for all; if you are a Full Hourglass or a Round, avoid the center crease.

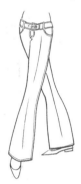

**Bootleg** Helps balance full hips on Triangles and Full Hourglasses.

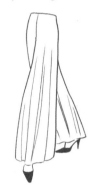

**Palazzo** Avoid the very wide styles if you are short-legged. Make sure the length is right.

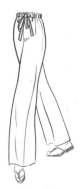

**Drawstring** Good for fluctuating waistlines and for comfort in a more casual look.

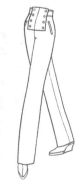

**High waistband** Good for Lean Columns and those who are long-bodied with narrow hips.

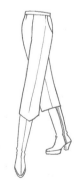

**Cropped** Make sure these finish at a narrow point on your calf. Avoid cuffs if legs are short.

# dresses

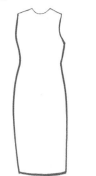

**Straight sheath** Best on Lean Columns, Rectangles, and Inverted Triangles.

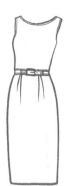

**Fitted, belted sheath** This shaped sheath is ideal for Neat and Full Hourglasses.

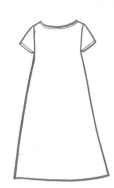

**A-line** A great look for Rounds, but avoid if you are a Triangle and have full hips.

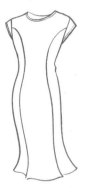

**Princess line** Great for Neat and Full Hourglasses, since it shows off the body shape.

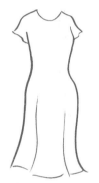

**Bias cut** Curves are essential for this shape, so good for Neat and Full Hourglasses and Triangles.

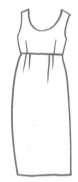

**Empire line** A good style to break up a long body and for expectant moms.

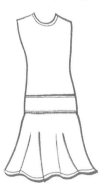

**Dropped waist** This style will work for those of you who are high-waisted.

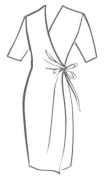

**Wrap** A winner on Neat and Full Hourglass shapes and expectant moms.

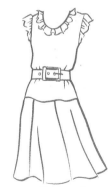

**Separates** The perfect combination for Triangles, Inverted Triangles, and Rounds.

# proportions

WHEN YOU LOOK AT PROPORTIONS, YOU ARE CONSIDERING THE RELATIONSHIP OF YOUR BODY TO YOUR LEGS, AS WELL AS THE POSITION OF YOUR WAIST. ONCE YOU UNDERSTAND YOUR BODY PROPORTIONS, YOU'LL BE ABLE TO COMBINE CLOTHES THAT APPEAR TO ADJUST ANY IMBALANCES AND GIVE THE ILLUSION OF PERFECT PROPORTIONS.

## the possible combinations

High-waisted + short rise + long legs
High-waisted + long rise + average to short legs
Low-waisted + short rise + average to short legs
Low-waisted + long rise + short legs
Balanced waist + balanced rise + balanced legs

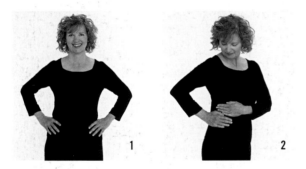

Stand in front of a mirror so that you can see your silhouette. Place your hands on your natural waistline (1). Then place the palm of one hand underneath your bust, and the other below the first hand (2). If you can easily place two hands widthways between your bust and waistline, you are low-waisted and may be slightly shorter in the leg. If you have to struggle to get the second hand in, you have long legs and may be high-waisted. If you can get approximately 1½ hands in, you have perfect proportions. You may feel that you have a large bottom, but it could be that you are long in the rise.

## BALANCED WAIST

**Balanced rise + legs**
You are extremely lucky to have perfect proportions, with the length of your body and legs in balance with each other. Remember what your height, scale, and body shape are and follow the guidelines given in the appropriate section of this book (pages 110–129) whenever you go clothes shopping. This will guarantee that you only buy what suits you the best.

## HIGH-WAISTED

### Short rise + long legs

Create the illusion of lowering your waist:

- Dropped waistlines or low-rise pants.
- Skirts and pants without waistbands.
- Low-slung belts.
- Long jackets and tops.
- Volume or pattern on your legs.
- Long tops and long skirts.
- Don't tuck in tops.

### Long rise + average to short legs

Create the illusion of lowering your waist without shortening your legs:

- Low waistlines or low-rise pants.
- Skirts and pants without waistbands.
- Low-slung belts.
- High heels.
- Long jackets and tops with narrow skirts or pants.
- Don't clutter your leg area.
- Don't tuck in tops.

## LOW-WAISTED

### Short rise + average to short legs

Create the illusion of raising your waist without shortening your legs:

- Belts and tuck-ins.
- Short tops.
- Minimal details in the rise area.
- Short jackets with long or short skirts.
- Straight-waisted or belted dresses.
- Long jackets with short skirts or narrow pants.
- High heels.
- Don't clutter your leg area.

### Long rise + short legs

Create the illusion of raising your waist and lengthening your legs:

- Belts and tuck-ins.
- Short tops and jackets.
- Details such as pockets or trims in the rise area.
- Stick to one color from waist to toe.
- High heels.
- Straight-waisted or belted dresses.
- Don't clutter your leg area.

# scale

SCALE IS A COMBINATION OF HEIGHT AND BONE STRUCTURE. YOUR SCALE MAY BE PETITE, AVERAGE, OR GRAND, AND WILL DETERMINE THE SIZE OF PATTERNS, THE WEIGHT OF FABRICS, AND HOW MUCH TEXTURE YOU CAN WEAR, AS WELL AS THE SIZE OF YOUR ACCESSORIES.

## PETITE

**5FT 3IN (1.6M) AND UNDER**
- You're better wearing one color from head to toe
- Two colors may be worn as long as the proportions are ⅔ to ⅓
- Best not to wear too much volume—it will swamp you

### SCALE
You have:
- fine fingers, narrow wrists and ankles
- small facial features
- shoe size under 6½

### YOU SHOULD WEAR:
- smaller print patterns
- smaller accessories
- minimal texture and bulk
- neat hairstyles

## AVERAGE

**5FT 3IN–5FT 7IN (1.6–1.7M)**
- You have the freedom to do what you like, as long as you follow your body shape (pages 112–129) and proportions (pages 136–137)

### SCALE
You have:
- neither petite nor grand bone structure
- shoe size between 6½ and 9

### YOU SHOULD WEAR:
- accessories that will balance your scale (neither tiny nor extra-large)
- average-sized patterns
- either a "wow" piece of clothing to make a statement or a single accessory such as a bag or a piece of jewelry

## GRAND

**5FT 7IN (1.7M) AND OVER**
- You need to use color to break up your height
- By wearing differently proportioned clothes you will look more balanced (short jacket + short skirt will not do)

### SCALE
You have:
- large hands and feet, and strong bone structure
- shoe size 9+

### YOU SHOULD WEAR:
- larger, bolder prints
- statement accessories
- heavier-weighted fabrics (or finer fabrics worn layered)

# flattering color combinations

NOW THAT YOU KNOW YOUR BEST COLORS, YOU CAN COMBINE THEM TO CREATE THE LOOK OF A BALANCED BODY. LIGHTER OR BRIGHTER COLORS WILL ALWAYS DRAW ATTENTION TO THE AREAS WHERE THEY'RE WORN. BELOW ARE SOME OF THE MOST FREQUENTLY USED COMBINATIONS.

## ALL-OVER COLOR

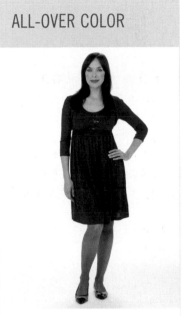

One color used for the entire outfit, or a single-colored dress, will give the appearance of height.

## COLOR BLOCKS

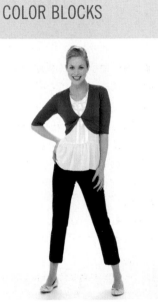

Different blocks of color on a jacket, top, skirt, or pants will give the appearance of reducing height.

## TWO COLORS

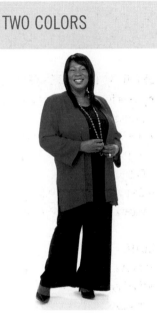

A jacket and skirt or pants in one color, with a top of another color, is a great combination for everybody.

## OTHER WINNING COMBINATIONS

- A light top with a dark bottom will give the illusion of wider shoulders and slimmer hips, which is perfect for Triangles, but not for Inverted Triangles.
- A jacket in one color, with a top and skirt or pants in another, is a great combination for every body shape. If you are long in the body, you can break this look up with a belt.
- A dark top and light bottom will give the illusion of narrower shoulders and wider hips. This combination is excellent for Inverted Triangles, but not for Triangles; you need a light top and a darker bottom.

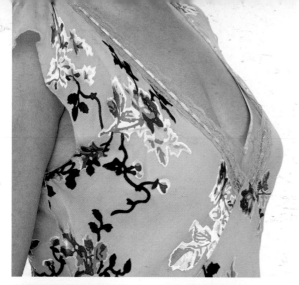

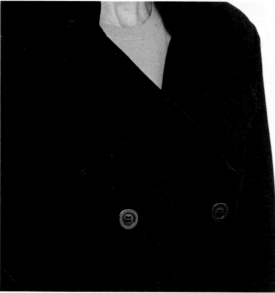

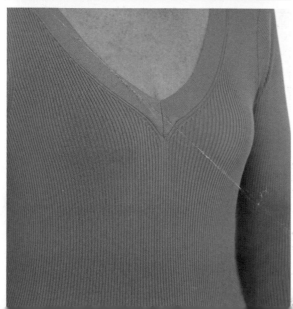

# clothing details

YOUR BODY SHAPE AND PROPORTIONS WILL
DETERMINE WHICH CLOTHING DETAILS, SUCH AS
NECKLINES, WAISTLINES, AND SLEEVES, WILL FLATTER
YOU THE MOST. BY LEARNING TO LOOK AT YOUR BODY
OBJECTIVELY, YOU WILL KNOW HOW TO BUY CLOTHES
TO SUIT YOUR SHAPE.

## the golden rule

There is one golden rule that will ensure that you
are showing off your body shape to best advantage
at all times: **never finish any part of a garment
at the widest point of your body**. For example,
you should avoid:
- jackets that finish at the widest point on your hips
- skirts that end at the fullest part of your legs
- short sleeves if you have a full bust
- short tops if you have a wide waist

## bustlines

If you don't wear the right bra, your clothes won't
hang properly: *go to page 180*—the wrong bra can
affect your body shape and clothing size. Have a
variety of bras to wear on different occasions and
with different tops.
**Small bust** Add details such as pockets, buttons,
appliqué, ruffles, or slogans. Texture and layering
are also helpful. A padded bra always helps.
**Full bust** Stick to simple cuts and plain fabrics
(no heavy textures). A V-neck or jewel neckline is
best for you. Front-opening shirts and blouses
need to be worn with care, and should be made
of soft or stretchy fabric.

# necklines

When deciding which necklines to wear, be aware of how prominent your collarbones and/or your upper chest are, and of how confident you feel about revealing these parts of your body.

**Boat/slash** Give the illusion of wide shoulders. Good for Triangle shapes, but avoid if you have prominent collarbones or a scrawny neck.

**Bardot** Good for most shapes, but not if you have sloping shoulders.

**V-necks** Look good on everyone, and can always be accessorized. Plunging V-necks are elegant—but not if you have a long neck or if they reveal too much cleavage.

**Scoop** Work well on most women, particularly if you have narrow shoulders.

**Cowl** Perfect for full busts and softer body lines.

**Turtle** Only if you have a long neck and no double chin or short neck.

**Crew** Suit most women, but they need to sit well.

**Ruffles/frills** Best for a longer neck and softer facial features.

**Mandarin collars** Not for those with a short neck or double chin.

**Shirt collars** Good for most women (unless short-necked), and best worn open.

**Jewel necklines** Good for all.

**Halter necks** Excellent for Inverted Triangles.

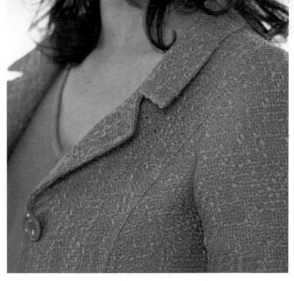

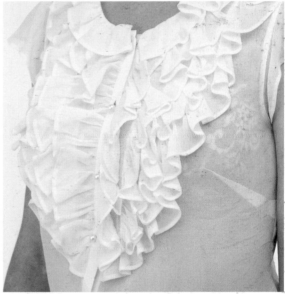

# shoulder lines

**Inset** Good for all. If your shoulders slope or are rounded, consider shoulder pads.

**Raglan** You need a square shoulder line to wear these successfully.

**Dropped** Good for adding width to the shoulders. They will also soften a strong, straight shoulder line.

**Shoulder pads** Great for straightening out sloping shoulders.

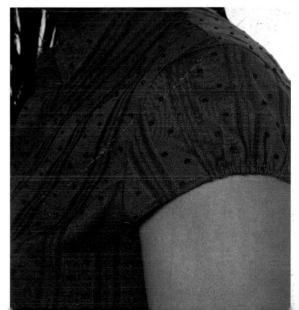

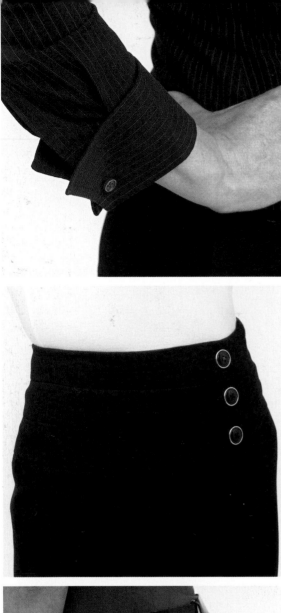

## sleeves

The key factor when choosing a sleeve length is to remember never to end the sleeves at a wide point on your arm.

**Bracelet** Great for short to average arms.
**Full** Best for average to long arms.
**Batwing** Best worn by average to tall women.
**Cuff details** Make sure these do not overwhelm your hands.

## waistlines

Create the illusion of a longer body by wearing a low waistline; to shorten your body, bring the waistline up.

**Waistband** You need to have a clearly defined waist, as in Neat Hourglass, Full Hourglass, and Triangle shapes, to wear pants and skirts with waistbands. A wide waistband is excellent if you are long-waisted.

**Elasticized** These may be your favorites if you have a fluctuating waistline. Best worn covered over, but beware of adding bulk. Nongathered elasticized waistbands are more flattering.

**Dropped waist** Perfect for short-waisted women, but they don't work well for long-waisted women.

**Low-rise** Good for short waists and those of you who do not have clearly defined waistlines (Inverted Triangles, Rectangles, or Lean Columns).

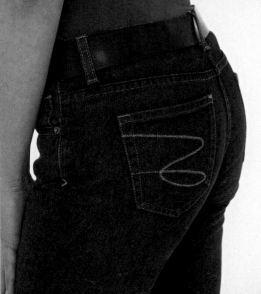

## bottom lines

Decide where the widest part of your bottom is and avoid any details in that area. Instead of wearing a long jacket or top to hide your bottom, show off an asset such as your waist.

## tummy lines

**Front pleats** Good if you have a flat tummy.

**Zippers** Front zippers will add volume to your tummy; side and back zippers will give a sleeker look.

**Pockets** Pockets with flaps suit women with flat hips. Sloping pockets and pockets without flaps can be worn by everyone.

**Belts** Great for averting the eye from a full, rounded tummy.

## thigh lines

If your thighs are wider than your hips, be careful to avoid details in the thigh area. Looser-fitting pants and skirts are the answer.

## leg lines

**Short legs** Wear skirts and pants with minimal volume. Open-fronted shoes with a short skirt will add length to the leg, as will hose or socks in the same color as your pants or skirt. Avoid details and patterns.

**Long legs** Wear skirts and pants with lots of volume and detail. Patterns and layers are good for you.

**Skinny legs** Add volume with textured hose and fabrics. Avoid anything too clingy.

**Wide legs** Wear the same color from waist to toes. Avoid anything too clingy or heavily textured. Loose and fluid fits work well.

## ankle lines

**Thin** Add details such as ankle straps, socks, or different textures.

**Wide** Go for open-fronted shoes.

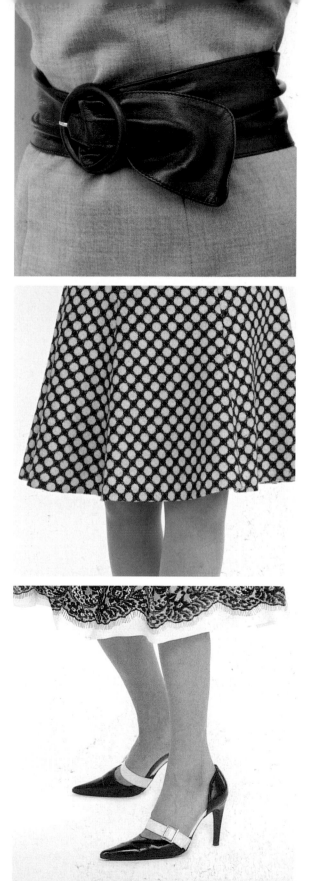

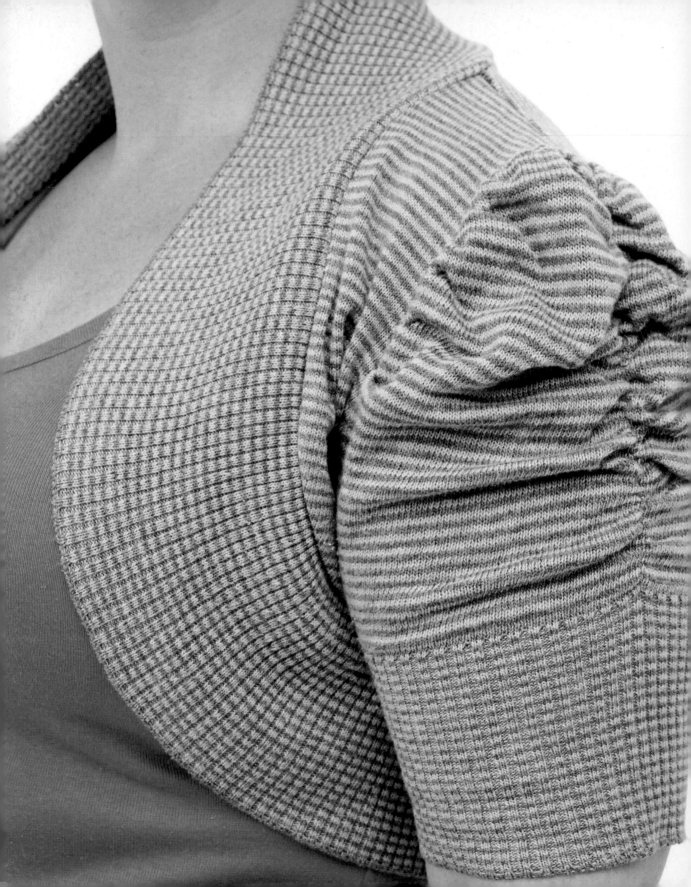

# 4

# finding your style

# your style personality

NATURALLY, THE COLOR AND STYLING OF YOUR CLOTHES PLAY AN IMPORTANT PART IN YOUR APPEARANCE, BUT IT IS YOUR PERSONALITY THAT ACTS AS A CATALYST AND PULLS YOUR WHOLE LOOK TOGETHER. YOUR PERSONALITY DICTATES YOUR STYLE, WHICH IS YOUR OWN INTERPRETATION OF FASHION AND HOW YOU LIKE TO WEAR CLOTHES.

Once you know and understand your style personality, putting your wardrobe together will become second nature. If you ignore your personality and buy clothes simply because they're featured in all the glossy magazines or look great on a friend, you will not look comfortable and your wardrobe will be a mishmash of styles. This, in turn, will limit your flexibility in mixing and matching to create the perfect outfits for you. It also means that you won't get the best value from your clothing investments.

The clothes you wear and how you wear them are governed by many factors: age, build, lifestyle, environment, budget, culture, and personal preferences. The way you project yourself may be influenced by your upbringing, the way you want others to see you, or even by a misguided approach to how you see yourself. Knowing your style personality will give you the foundation on which to project yourself in a more organized way, and to feel comfortable in your outfit, whatever the occasion.

## styles of the famous

Before determining your own style personality, take a look at how famous people dress. Notice what they are wearing when they appear to be at their most comfortable and relaxed.

Singer Gwen Stefani is a true **Creative**, changing her look constantly to suit her latest record or video. A trendsetter rather than a trend follower, she loves avant-garde designers.

Television celebrity Sharon Osbourne has a **Dramatic** style personality, choosing clothes that get her noticed and sometimes even shock. She loves setting trends and working with the latest designers to create a look that's new and different.

With her wonderful long, wavy hair, actress Nicole Kidman epitomizes the **Romantic** style personality. Away from the red carpet, she loves pretty, feminine details and luxury fabrics.

Former Secretary of State Condoleezza Rice is an example of the **Classic** style personality. Her look is the same every time she is seen in public: simple and groomed. Nothing is out of place, nothing shocks, and she is completely coordinated.

Dame Ellen MacArthur, British yachtswoman, has a **Natural** style personality. She doesn't care about the world seeing her unkempt, with messy hair and without any makeup.

Actress Catherine Deneuve has developed an elegance that is fashionable but not trendy. Her clothes are understated and her accessories always in vogue. It's difficult to recall exactly what she wears—you just remember that she looks good, and this is the key factor of **City Chic** style.

## changing your style

As you progress though life, you will feel different about the way you look. What you wear in your early twenties, for example, will be very different from how you will want to dress when middle-aged or later in life.

*Knowing your style personality will enable you to feel comfortable in your outfit, whatever the occasion*

In your teens you might flaunt your body by wearing revealing outfits, or follow fashion fads regardless of whether they suit you. You might find yourself going out of your way to shock others with what you wear, or you may show no interest at all in clothes, personal grooming, shopping, or accessories.

As you begin to think about attracting the opposite sex, your clothes can become an extension of your sexuality. You may start to wear makeup or apply more than you used to. You may even wear really uncomfortable items of clothing simply because they help you convey how you feel inside. If you feel romantic, you may portray that emotion on the outside by wearing feminine clothes. Floral patterns may creep into your wardrobe, fabrics may become sheerer, and you may wear the occasional frilly number.

As you advance in your career or become a parent, you may feel that you need a more classic look, and that you should put on a "uniform" to match your new status in life. You start to think about making your clothes last for more than one season. Expensive investment purchases now

feature in your wardrobe, and you consider how versatile an item might be before you buy it.

There are, of course, those of you who simply enjoy clothes—you're not fashion victims, but you like to look up to date. You have experimented over the years and have discovered what suits you, and probably have some basic items that form the core of your look. You enjoy shopping for accessories and special pieces to enhance your wardrobe. Through good advice or experimentation, you will have already learned what does and what doesn't work for you.

Some of you will have been through all these various style stages, and may feel that you are stuck in a format that's comfortable but boring. Now is the time to move on and try something new and different.

## identifying your look

Completing the questionnaire on the next two pages will help you determine your style personality. Some of you will discover that you have a split style personality, and you will need to decide which one is the most appropriate for you, although it is possible to be one type for work and another for socializing.

Those of you who are really adept at planning your wardrobe might be a little of all of the personalities, depending on the occasion and how you feel at any particular time.

Keep in mind that there is also a psychological aspect to color and the colors you wear: *go to pages 28–31*.

# style personality questionnaire

TO FIND OUT YOUR STYLE PERSONALITY, COMPLETE THE QUESTIONNAIRE BELOW, CIRCLING AS MANY OPTIONS AS YOU WISH. YOU MAY FEEL THAT SOME QUESTIONS MERIT MORE THAN ONE ANSWER—FOR EXAMPLE, ONE MAY DESCRIBE HOW YOU DRESS DURING THE WEEK, ANOTHER MAY REFLECT YOUR APPEARANCE ON WEEKENDS, AND A THIRD MAY DESCRIBE HOW YOU WOULD LIKE TO LOOK. TAKE THE PLUNGE AND DISCOVER THE REAL YOU!

## HOW DO YOU WEAR COLOR?

- **A** Whatever I feel like on the day.
- **B** Strong, contrasting and bright shades.
- **C** Pretty pastels.
- **D** I like to be coordinated.
- **E** I go for simple color combinations.
- **F** A tone-on-tone look.

## WHAT KIND OF SHOPPER ARE YOU?

- **A** I love flea markets and vintage clothes.
- **B** I buy something if I like it.
- **C** I enjoy the whole shopping experience.
- **D** I plan my shopping trips and take a list.
- **E** I buy when I need something.
- **F** I am an investment buyer.

## HOW WOULD YOU DESCRIBE YOUR OVERALL LOOK?

- **A** Eclectic and sometimes wacky.
- **B** I like to make a statement and wear eye-catching pieces.
- **C** Pretty, with detailed clothes that make me feel feminine.
- **D** Neat, organized, and coordinated.
- **E** Relaxed and casual.
- **F** Simple and elegant.

## WHAT IS IN YOUR WORKING WARDROBE?

- **A** Individual pieces.
- **B** Eye-catching pieces.
- **C** Pretty blouses and tops that I combine with a jacket.
- **D** Tailored suits.
- **E** Easy-to-wear separates.
- **F** Basic pieces, but dressed up with accessories.

## WHAT IS IN YOUR NONWORKING WARDROBE?

- **A** My collection of vintage clothes.
- **B** My latest fashion purchase.
- **C** Pretty, feminine pieces.
- ⊙ **D** Coordinated separates.
- **E** Jeans and comfortable tops.
- **F** Simple styles, which I accessorize.

## WHAT IS IN YOUR SPECIAL OCCASION WARDROBE?

- **A** Velvet, brocade, antiques, and lace.
- **B** Unusual and striking garments.
- **C** Fitted dresses with lots of detailing.
- **D** Simple and tailored dresses.
- ⊙ **E** Comfortable, dressy pants or a long skirt with a loose-fitting top.
- **F** An elegant dress or pantsuit.

## WHAT ARE YOUR SHOES LIKE?

- **A** They don't coordinate with my outfit.
- **B** High-heeled or funky.
- **C** Pretty, with bows and details.
- **D** They match my handbag.
- ⊙ **E** Comfortable.
- **F** Current.

## WHAT KIND OF JEWELRY DO YOU LIKE?

- **A** Unusual—I collect it.
- **B** Bold, makes a statement.
- **C** Intricate, dangly and pretty.
- **D** Simple and fine.
- ⊙ **E** Minimal.
- **F** Current and noticeable.

## WHAT IS YOUR ATTITUDE TO MAKEUP?

- **A** I experiment.
- **B** I like it to be noticed.
- **C** I love it and spend time over it.
- ⊙ **D** I keep to the same routine.
- **E** Minimalistic.
- **F** It complements my look.

## WHAT TYPE OF HAIRSTYLE DO YOU HAVE?

- **A** It changes with my mood.
- **B** It changes regularly.
- **C** Long.
- ⊙ **D** Neat.
- ⊙ **E** Low maintenance.
- **F** Up to date.

## YOUR RESULTS

Once you have completed the questionnaire, count how many times you have answered A, B and so on, and see right to determine your predominant style personality. Then refer to the following pages for examples of famous people who match your style personality and for tips on how to achieve the style.

**Mainly A**  Creative: **go to pages 150–151**
**Mainly B**  Dramatic: **go to pages 152–153**
**Mainly C**  Romantic: **go to pages 154–155**
**Mainly D**  Classic: **go to pages 156–157**
**Mainly E**  Natural: **go to pages 158–159**
**Mainly F**  City Chic: **go to pages 160–161**

# creative

YOU ARE GREAT AT COMBINING DIFFERENT ITEMS OF CLOTHING AND ACCESSORIES TO GIVE YOURSELF A UNIQUE AND INTERESTING LOOK, AND YOU RARELY THROW ANYTHING OUT BECAUSE YOU KNOW YOU WILL USE IT AT SOME POINT, EVEN IF IT HAS TO BE REMODELED. IF YOU'RE NOT CAREFUL, THOUGH, YOUR CREATIVE TENDENCIES COULD RESULT IN YOUR BEING INAPPROPRIATELY DRESSED FOR CERTAIN OCCASIONS.

## FAMOUS CREATIVES

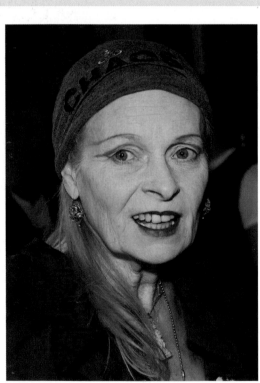

Vivienne Westwood (pictured)

Helena Bonham Carter

Kate Moss

Cher

Gwen Stefani

## style characteristics

- Your wardrobe is full of items from many different sources, including vintage mixed with high fashion, that you have collected over the years.
- For you, shopping is an art form. You like nothing better than rummaging around a thrift store or your mother's attic. You find chain stores distasteful and boring.
- You often make interesting purchases while on vacation, and look at fashion magazines for inspiration and ideas.

## make the most of your style

- Team chunky knits with floaty dresses and funky boots.
- Wear pants with tunics and dresses, teamed with a low-slung belt.
- Make office wear more interesting with an eye-catching blouse or a scarf, mixed with unusual accessories.
- For the evening, choose a vintage dress, perhaps with a pair of jeweled shoes.

# your color palette

**Light** Primrose + light aqua, geranium + blush pink, light navy + apple green.

**Deep** Chocolate + eggplant, taupe + royal purple, lime + turquoise.

**Warm** Tangerine + mint, purple + bittersweet, charcoal + oatmeal.

**Cool** Light periwinkle + hot pink, duck egg + teal, blue-red + icy green.

**Clear** Black + apple green, light apricot + royal blue, ruby + light teal.

**Soft** Shell + soft violet, claret + rose brown, sage + charcoal blue.

# how to accessorize

- Choose a belt that will make a statement.
- Wear a scarf that doesn't coordinate with or match what you are wearing.
- Add costume jewelry or interesting ethnic pieces as finishing touches.
- Customize clothes with interesting buttons.
- Add a corsage or pin to a vintage jacket to bring it up to date.
- Wear a hat, no matter what the weather's like.

# your face

**Day** Choose either your eyes or your lips to create a wow effect with makeup.

**Evening** Combine colors that do not necessarily match what you are wearing.

# your hair

Add outrageous colors to your hair. Accessorize with unusual combs, barrettes, flowers, and scarves. Experiment with braids and hair extensions.

# dramatic

YOU ALWAYS WANT TO MAKE AN ENTRANCE. YOU LOVE TO BE NOTICED AND OFTEN WEAR CLOTHES WITH A WOW FACTOR. WHATEVER THE LATEST FASHION, YOU WILL GIVE IT A TRY, EVEN IF IT DOESN'T PARTICULARLY SUIT YOU. SHOPPING IS ONE OF YOUR FAVORITE PASTIMES. YOU LIKE TO PARTY—SPENDING A QUIET EVENING AT HOME READING A BOOK IS NOT YOUR THING.

## FAMOUS DRAMATICS

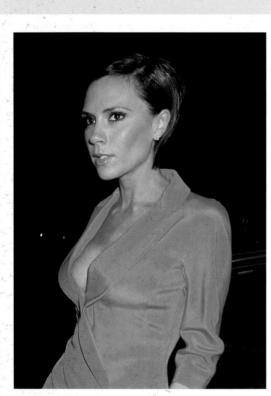

**Victoria Beckham**
(pictured)
**Madonna**
**Naomi Campbell**

**Sharon Osbourne**
**Donatella Versace**
**Shilpa Shetty**

## style characteristics

- Your wardrobe consists of many different styles of clothes and individual pieces that you have bought on impulse, without a thought as to whether you have anything to wear with them.
- Your friends are often envious of your striking appearance and style.
- You are not concerned with whether your clothes are practical or washable—they just have to make a statement.
- You will scour the fashion press for the latest trends and ideas.

## make the most of your style

- Wear separates in contrasting colors.
- The bolder and more striking your accessories, the better.
- In the evening, wear that "Oscar" dress; it's your style to dress up, rather than down, for parties and special occasions.
- Be prepared to tone down your look for the daytime in the office.

## your color palette

**Light** Light gray + geranium, peacock + blush pink, taupe + violet.

**Deep** Black + soft white, scarlet + damson, chocolate + fern.

**Warm** Purple + amber, bronze + daffodil, orange-red + aqua.

**Cool** Charcoal + periwinkle, cassis + royal blue, spruce + blue-green.

**Clear** True blue + ivory, apple green + light apricot, true red + black-brown.

**Soft** Purple + light periwinkle, emerald turquoise + mint, rose brown + claret.

## how to accessorize

- Wear belts with interesting buckles and details, such as studs, jewels, or cut-out patterns.
- Make a statement with bold patterns in contrasting colors.
- Wear large, striking jewelry, but not too much at once.
- Update your look each season with new shoes or boots.
- Throw a colorful scarf over your winter coat.
- Always wear a hat or hair accessory.

## your face

**Day** Don't forget your eye pencil plus two or three coats of mascara, and your lip gloss.

**Evening** Nothing but the full works for you, finished off with a red lipstick.

## your hair

Add a striking color to your hair (in tones that complement your coloring). Change your hairstyle regularly and consult your hairdresser to keep up with the latest styles. Use hair treatments and styling products to keep your hair in top condition at all times.

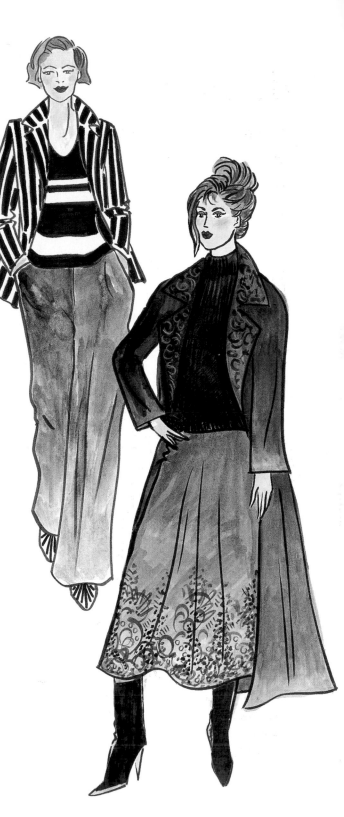

# romantic

YOU LOVE EVERYTHING ABOUT DRESSING UP AND PLANNING YOUR WARDROBE. YOUR CLOTHES ARE PRETTY, AND YOU ADORE ALL SORTS OF DETAILS: BOWS, RUFFLES, FLOUNCES, APPLIQUÉS, AND FRINGES. YOU LOVE TO EXPERIMENT WITH NEW SKINCARE AND BODYCARE PRODUCTS, AND NEVER GO OUT WITHOUT YOUR PERFUME. YOU WILL SPEND LONGER THAN ANYBODY ELSE LOOKING AFTER YOURSELF AND YOUR GROOMING.

## FAMOUS ROMANTICS

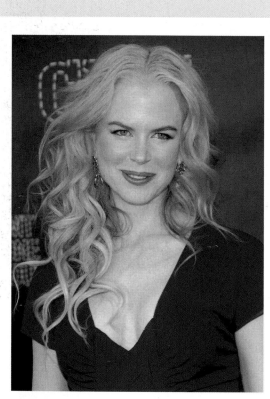

Nicole Kidman (pictured)
Sarah Ferguson,
   Duchess of York
Elizabeth Hurley

Scarlett Johansson
Penelope Cruz
Charlize Theron

## style characteristics

- Flowers feature heavily in your wardrobe, whether in patterned fabrics or as accessories and decorative details, such as corsages, pins, and other jewelry.
- You always wear matching and pretty underwear, even if it is uncomfortable.
- Your sports clothes are either in pretty colors or have decorative details.
- Even your business clothes are pretty, feminine, and detailed.

## make the most of your style

- Choose separates that are decorated with beading, appliqué, or ribbons.
- Choose luxury fabrics such as angora, cashmere, silk, and satin.
- Skirts or dresses teamed with a cardigan or pretty jacket are a great look for you.
- In the evening, go for a layered look and choose fabrics such as chiffon or lace decorated with sequins and rhinestones. Complete the look with high-heeled sandals.

## your color palette

**Light** Light navy + pastel pink, pewter + mint, light aqua + light apricot.

**Deep** Charcoal + blush pink, cornflower + primrose, eggplant + moss.

**Warm** Coral + cream, gray-green + teal, amber + taupe.

**Cool** Rose pink + baby pink, sky blue + medium gray, bright periwinkle + icy green.

**Clear** Emerald turquoise + duck egg, scarlet + light gray, royal blue + light apricot.

**Soft** Blush pink + soft violet, spruce + mint, cocoa + shell.

## how to accessorize

- Add a flower somewhere: in your hair, on your shoulder, to your bag, or even to your shoes.
- Floral prints work well if you have soft body lines; if you don't, choose polka dots or squiggles.
- Wear dangling, detailed jewelry.
- Decorative handbags are perfect for you.
- Wear fine patterned or textured hose; seamed stockings are fun if you have shapely legs and ankles.
- Always wear a heel, whether on a sandal or boot.

## your face

**Day** You always wear makeup, especially a pink lipstick and a blush from your palette.

**Evening** For an ultrafeminine look, dazzle with sparkle, shimmer, and glitter.

## your hair

The best hairstyles for you are long and layered, softly curled, and probably highlighted. Put decorations in your hair if you wear it up.

# classic

YOU HAVE A FAIRLY FORMAL WARDROBE. YOU LIKE TO APPEAR WELL TURNED OUT AND ELEGANT, AND YOUR TOPS ARE USUALLY TUCKED IN. YOU ARE HAPPY TO STAY WITH THE SAME HAIRSTYLES, AND HATE IT WHEN YOUR HAIRDRESSER MOVES AWAY. YOUR MAKEUP ROUTINE IS FIXED, AND YOU RARELY EXPERIMENT WITH NEW SHADES. YOU HAVE A FEW FAVORITE STORES THAT YOU VISIT WHEN YOU NEED NEW CLOTHES.

## FAMOUS CLASSICS

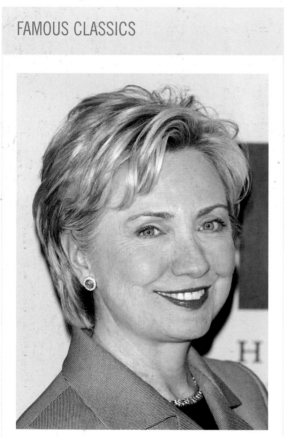

Hillary Clinton (pictured)   Condoleezza Rice
Laura Bush                   Martha Stewart
Martina Navratilova          Angela Merkel
Princess Anne

## style characteristics

- Your look is timeless and elegant.
- You prefer a coordinated look and do not like to mix textures or wear daring color combinations.
- Your workwear is tasteful and understated; you only ever wear pattern on scarves.
- On weekends you are likely to replace your jacket and blouse with a twinset.
- You rarely wear jeans, preferring a pair of classic pants teamed with leather loafers.
- You do not follow fashion.

## make the most of your style

- Coordinated separates are the basis of all your looks.
- By mixing and matching what you already have, you will create many more outfits.
- Add colored tops to your basic jackets to achieve a more varied look.
- Your evening wear will be simple, to which you will add your favorite pieces of jewelry.

## your color palette

**Light** Stone + cornflower, light navy + dusty rose, cocoa + light aqua.

**Deep** Charcoal + burgundy, black–brown + moss, pewter + teal.

**Warm** Gray-green + oatmeal, chocolate + cream, bronze + amber.

**Cool** Dark navy + icy blue, pine + light teal, medium gray + rose pink.

**Clear** Black + duck egg, dark navy + emerald turquoise, taupe + blush pink.

**Soft** Natural beige + verbena, charcoal blue + shell, chocolate + mint.

## how to accessorize

- Match your belt, handbag, and shoes.
- A scarf will always finish your look.
- Add quality costume jewelry to the real thing to create a more varied look.
- The quickest way for you to update your look is with a new pair of shoes in the latest style.
- Change your handbag regularly.
- Do not wear all your favorite pieces of matching jewelry at the same time.

## your face

**Day** Don't be afraid to try some new eye shadow and lipstick colors once in a while.

**Evening** Go one or two tones darker within your colors.

## your hair

Consider changing your hairstyle every two or three years, keeping your color as close to your natural shade as possible. Your preferred styles are easy to manage without complicated styling techniques.

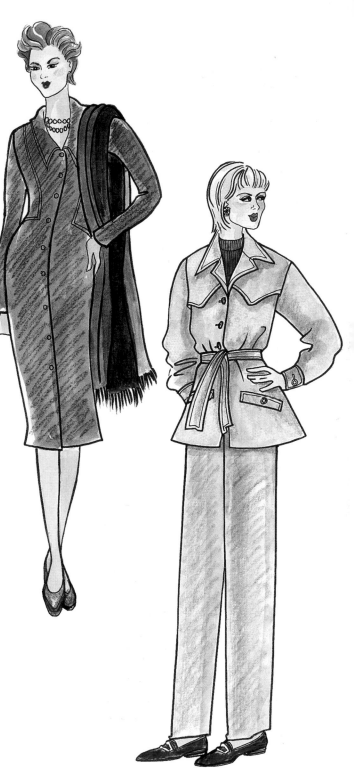

# natural

FEELING COMFORTABLE IN YOUR CLOTHES IS THE MOST IMPORTANT FACTOR FOR YOU WHEN CHOOSING WHAT TO WEAR; ANYTHING THAT CONSTRICTS, DIGS IN, OR PINCHES IS NOT AN OPTION. YOU PREFER CASUAL STYLING TO FORMAL BUSINESS WEAR, AND YOU HATE A CLUTTERED LOOK—SIMPLE LINES AND DESIGNS ARE MORE YOU. IN KEEPING WITH YOUR NO-FUSS ATTITUDE, CLOTHES MUST BE EASY-CARE AND IDEALLY NONIRON.

## FAMOUS NATURALS

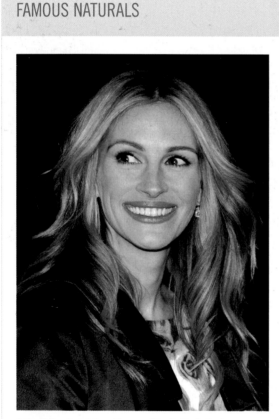

Julia Roberts (pictured)    Charlotte Gainsbourg
Steffi Graf                 Vanessa Redgrave
Lauren Hutton               Kate Winslet

## style characteristics

- Your closet may appear disorganized, and you will often just wear whatever is on hand and clean that morning.
- Pants worn with flat shoes are your preference for maximum comfort and practicality.
- You have many interests, but reading fashion magazines is not one of them.
- Your jewelry will be minimal—if you wear any at all—and won't jangle.

## make the most of your style

- Long skirts—either full, pleated, or with a split—will allow freedom of movement; team them with boots or comfortable shoes.
- Go for deconstructed and loose-fitting clothes for a relaxed look.
- For work, comfort is still important, so choose a simple, good-quality top rather than a fussy, tailored shirt.
- For evening, try a tunic-type top over a pair of silk pants with flat pumps.

## your color palette

**Light** Stone + cornflower, medium gray + dusty rose, light navy + light aqua.

**Deep** Black + eggplant, dark navy + purple, stone + true red.

**Warm** Dark brown + terracotta, moss + cream, teal + turquoise.

**Cool** Rose beige + sapphire, pewter + bright periwinkle, pine + light gray.

**Clear** Black + evergreen, purple + lemon yellow, taupe + Chinese blue.

**Soft** Stone + claret, cocoa + jade, damson + shell.

## how to accessorize

- Your accessories will be minimal, but you still need them to complete your look.
- Wear a long scarf or pashmina over your coat or jacket, teamed with a pair of colorful gloves.
- For jewelry, choose natural materials such as wood, leather, and shell.
- A backpack-style handbag or one with a long shoulder strap is best for you.

## your face

**Day** Your makeup is minimal, so all-in-one products like tinted moisturizer are ideal.

**Evening** You don't tend to change your makeup dramatically for the evening; just add a fresh slick of a natural-colored lipstick or gloss.

## your hair

You don't like to spend much time on your tresses, so it's essential to have a good haircut that allows you to leave your hair to dry with little or no styling.

# city chic

YOU ENJOY YOUR CLOTHES BUT ARE NOT FANATICAL ABOUT THEM. YOU DEDICATE TIME AND THOUGHT TO THE WAY YOU LOOK, AND YOU LOVE ACCESSORIES, SOMETIMES SPENDING MORE ON BAGS AND SHOES THAN ON AN OUTFIT ITSELF. HAVING PROBABLY TRIED OUT MOST OF THE OTHER KEY STYLES AND EXPERIMENTED WITH LOTS OF DIFFERENT LOOKS, YOU NOW KNOW WHAT SUITS YOU.

## FAMOUS CITY CHICS

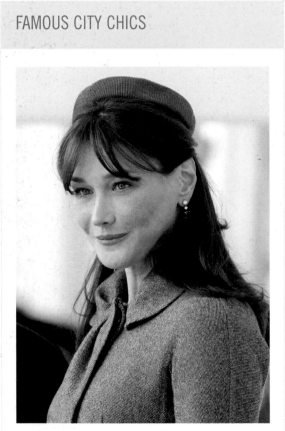

Carla Bruni-Sarkozy (pictured)

Catherine Deneuve

Honor Blackman

Isabella Rossellini

Sharon Stone

Oprah Winfrey

## style characteristics

- You tend to follow trends rather than mainstream fashion.
- You shop with care and rarely make rash purchases, ensuring that whatever you buy coordinates with other items that you already have in your wardrobe.
- You use bright colors with caution and tend to go for a tone-on-tone look.
- You keep abreast of the latest trends by reading good magazines.

## make the most of your style

- Invest in basic, classic pieces in neutral colors.
- Keep your working wardrobe updated with new tops, purchased regularly.
- Team pants with a stylish shirt or twin-set and accessorize appropriately.
- For evening, a simple sheath with a stunning necklace, worn with a colorful wrap or pashmina, will be a great success. Mules would be a good choice for footwear to complete this simple but stylish outfit.

## your color palette

**Light** Stone + cocoa, light periwinkle + sky blue, pastel pink + dusty rose.

**Deep** Black + charcoal, pine + mint, purple + damson.

**Warm** Bronze + moss, bittersweet + terracotta, daffodil + amber.

**Cool** Medium gray + light gray, light periwinkle + dark periwinkle, cassis + rose pink.

**Clear** True blue + royal blue, evergreen + emerald green, pewter + light teal.

**Soft** Cocoa + rose brown, sage + spruce, damson + soft violet.

## how to accessorize

- Make a statement with a single accessory, whether it is a stunning necklace, pin, or beaded scarf.
- Even when it's not sunny, always wear your sunglasses somewhere, such as on your head.
- Trade the black handbag for a colorful one.
- Tie a scarf to your handbag.
- Wear a quality watch.
- Wear an elegant heeled pump shoe with your slacks.

## your face

**Day** Create a matte finish for your face, and add a touch of bronzer and a neutral lipstick.

**Evening** Enhance your eye makeup with a granite or brown pencil, and add a little sheen or gloss to your eyelids; enhance your lips with a darker shade.

## your hair

Keep your hair in good condition and have it cut regularly. Subtle highlights and lowlights will give a natural look.

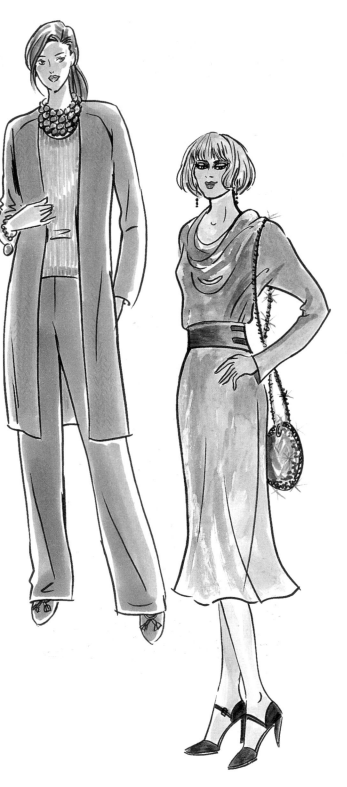

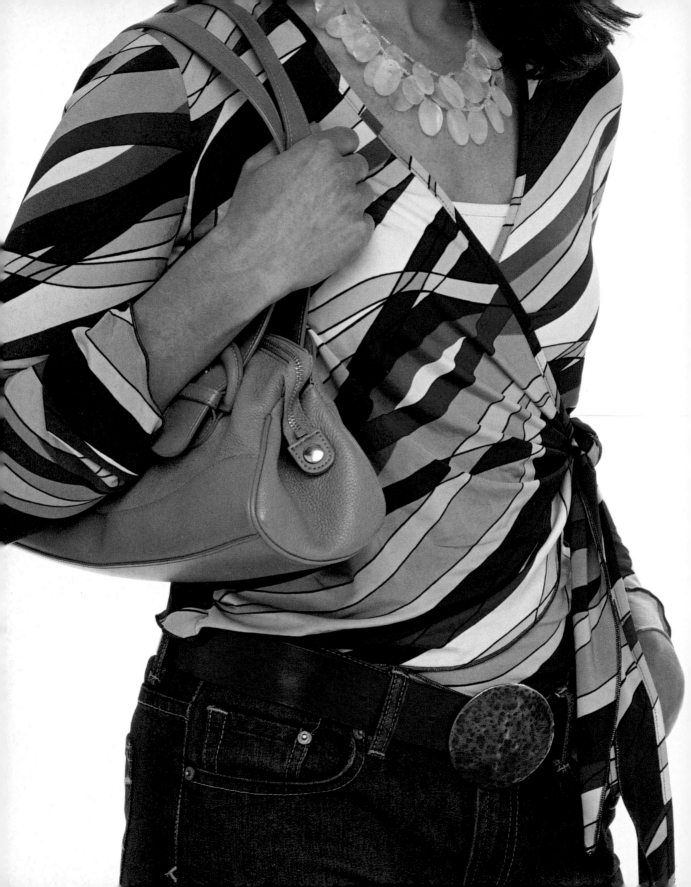

# 5

## pulling it all together

# face shape and proportion

NOW THAT YOU KNOW WHAT CLOTHES TO WEAR TO BEST COMPLEMENT YOUR COLORING, SHAPE, SIZE, AND STYLE, HERE'S HOW TO ADD THE FINISHING TOUCHES TO YOUR OUTFIT. THIS CHAPTER COVERS ALL THOSE ASPECTS YOU NEED TO CONSIDER TO PULL TOGETHER A COMPLETE LOOK, FROM YOUR HAIRSTYLE AND MAKEUP TO YOUR SHOES, AND EVERYTHING IN BETWEEN.

## DISCOVER YOUR FACE SHAPE

Even if you have a great figure and fabulous clothes, you won't look good if your hairstyle or eyeglasses don't work, your underwear is wrong, or your accessories ruin the outfit.

The first step is to discover your face shape. This will help you make informed choices about your hairstyle, makeup, glasses, and earrings.

The face is basically divided into three sections that should be evenly proportioned:

**Forehead to bridge of nose**
**Bridge of nose to base of nose**
**Base of nose to chin**

The optimum face shape is oval. This means:

**The widest point is at the cheekbones.**
**The face narrows gradually down to the jaw.**

## STEP 1—FACE SHAPE

- Tie or pin your hair back off your face.
- Wear a low neckline.
- Stand in front of a mirror.
- Using a water-soluble marker pen, draw the outline of your face onto the mirror.
- Stand back and look at the result.
- Is your basic face shape oval or round?
- Does your face have angles?
- Is the overall shape balanced?
- Does your face seem long?
- Is it wide at the top, narrowing down to a pointed chin?

## STEP 2—PROPORTIONS

- Standing in your original position, look at the outline of your face drawn on the mirror; mark the position of the bridge of your nose.
- Then draw another line at the base of your nose, and check the proportions (see above).

## STEP 3—PROFILE

- Turn to the side and look at your facial profile.
- Is there any feature that stands out disproportionately, such as your forehead, nose, or chin?

If your face shape and proportions are balanced, and you're happy with your profile, go straight to the page relating to your face shape. If not, read on to find out what to do.

# the challenges—proportions

### HIGH OR LOW FOREHEAD

The best way to minimize a high forehead is with bangs, whether full, layered, or asymmetric. If you have a low forehead, wear your hair off your face; if your hair naturally grows forward, ask your hairdresser to cut bangs from the top of your head—these are known as deep bangs—to give the illusion of a higher forehead.

### LONG NOSE

Use makeup to help create the illusion of a shorter nose. Highlight the nostril area with a light shade of foundation or concealer, and use a darker shade down the center of the nose. This will make the nose appear wider and shorter. Avoid a hairstyle with a center part.

### LONG CHIN

makeup can also help create the illusion of a shorter chin. Apply a foundation or concealer that is a shade darker than your normal one to the chin area, and use a lighter shade along the cheekbones to draw attention away from the chin.

# the challenges—profile

### LARGE NOSE

Apply a darker shade of foundation over the nose, and highlight the cheekbones with a lighter shade of foundation or concealer. Balance your profile with a hairstyle that adds volume to the back of your head—a hairstyle that is flat at the back will emphasize a large nose.

### DOUBLE CHIN

Use a darker powder, such as a bronzer, to cover the offending area (foundation will rub off on your clothes). To draw the eye away from the chin, emphasize your eyes or lips by using slightly brighter makeup. Anything around the neck, such as a high neckline, choker-type necklace, or scarf tied high, will draw attention to a double chin, so go for open necklines, longer necklaces, and loosely tied scarves.

### EARS THAT STICK OUT

Don't wear your hair tucked behind or cut around your ears—you need volume around and behind them. Avoid earrings that make a statement—they will draw attention to your ears.

## HOW TO CHOOSE EYEGLASSES

When you are choosing glasses, you need to consider your dominant color characteristics and your style personality, as well as your face shape and proportions. Check where the glasses sit on your nose: if you have a long nose, the bridge of the glasses should sit lower down to make your nose seem shorter; if you have a short nose, the bridge should sit higher. Your eyes should be in the center of the lenses. Think about having different styles for different occasions. For more advice on eyeglasses, see the relevant face shape: **go to pages 166–170.**

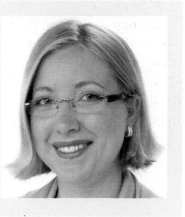

# oval

A BALANCED, OVAL FACE IS THE MOST VERSATILE FACE SHAPE AND GIVES YOU MANY OPTIONS
FOR HAIRSTYLES, MAKEUP, EYEGLASSES, AND EARRINGS, SINCE LOTS OF STYLES WILL SUIT YOU.
YOURS IS THE FACE SHAPE THAT EVERYONE WANTS TO HAVE.

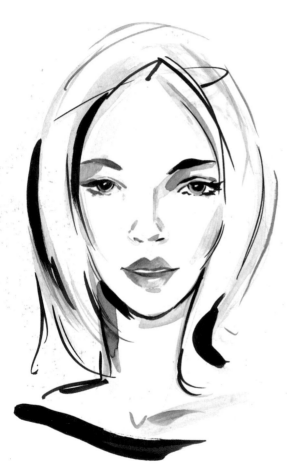

For more advice on applying makeup:
**go to pages 171–179.**

## makeup

**Eyebrows** Shape them so that they slant slightly
upwards at the end.
**Eye shadow** Use eye pencil and shadow to create
an almond-shaped eye: *go to page 176*.
**Blush** Follow the natural line of your cheekbones,
sweeping the brush upwards and outwards towards
the hairline.
**Lipstick** As long as your upper and lower lips are
balanced, follow your natural lip line.
**Top tip** Apply a hint of blush to the tip of the
chin and around the temples.

## hairstyle

Any style will complement an oval face shape, but
take into account your neck length, age, and hair
type. If you feel confident, wear your hair
completely swept away from your face.

## eyeglasses

Most shapes and styles will suit you, except
extreme geometric designs.

## earrings

If you have a short neck, you should avoid long,
chandelier-type earrings. Otherwise, you can wear
any style.

# square

YOU HAVE A WIDE FOREHEAD, AND YOUR CHEEKBONES ARE IN LINE WITH YOUR JAW. TO CREATE A MORE BALANCED FACE SHAPE, YOU CAN USE CLEVER SHADING TO SOFTEN THE SQUARENESS OF YOUR JAW AND EMPHASIZE YOUR CHEEKBONES.

## makeup

**Eyebrows** Shape your eyebrows to create a gentle arch above the center of each eye, directly over the pupil.

**Eye shadow** Apply highlighter under the center of the eyebrow and blend eye shadow, using upward strokes, towards the outer edge of the eye.

**Blush** Apply blush in a gently curved line along the cheekbones.

**Lipstick** Use a lip pencil to make your lips slightly fuller in the middle.

**Top tip** Apply darker shading (bronzer) on the edge of your jawline to soften the angle.

## hairstyle

Aim to add width to the upper part of your face, and soften the angles with curls or layers. Avoid straight bobs and heavy, straight bangs.

## eyeglasses

Look for lightweight oval or rounded frames. Avoid square or rectangular shapes, which will emphasize the angles of your face.

## earrings

Rounded shapes, such as hoops and ovals, are best; avoid sharp or angular designs.

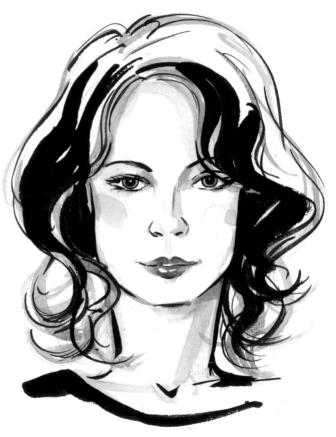

For more advice on applying makeup:
**go to pages 171–179.**

# rectangle

YOU HAVE A LONG, NARROW FACE WITH A SQUARISH CHIN. YOU NEED TO GIVE THE ILLUSION OF WIDENING AND SHORTENING THE FACE, WHILE SOFTENING THE JAWLINE. HORIZONTAL LINES MAKE THE FACE LOOK WIDER, SO EMPHASIZE YOUR EYEBROWS, CHEEKBONES, AND LIPS.

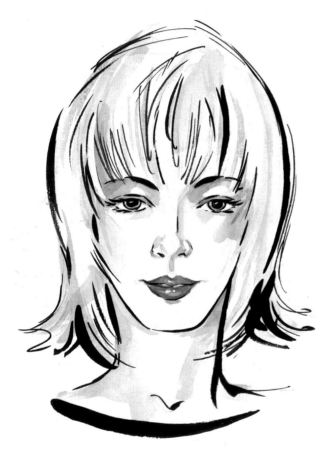

## makeup

**Eyebrows** Use a brow pencil to slightly extend the outer tails of your eyebrows, adding width.
**Eye shadow** Layer toning colors horizontally, working from the center of the eye outward.
**Blush** Follow the lines of your cheekbones, adding more definition near the hairline.
**Lipstick** Make your mouth look slightly wider when you line your lips with lip pencil, but keep it looking natural.
**Top tip** Apply a sweep of blush along the hair-line at cheekbone level to draw the eye outward.

## hairstyle

A layered style will help give the impression that your face is rounder and fuller. A softly layered crown is good, as is some fullness around the ear area. Bangs will also make your face appear shorter. Avoid long, straight styles with a center part—these will make your face look longer.

## eyeglasses

Lightweight, wider frames will counteract a narrow face and close-set eyes; avoid sharp, angular frames.

## earrings

Choose curvy shapes that add volume to your earlobes. Avoid long, dangly styles.

For more advice on applying makeup:
**go to pages 171–179.**

# inverted triangle

YOU HAVE A BROAD FOREHEAD AND CHEEKBONES, WHICH TAPER DOWN TO A SMALL CHIN. AIM
TO GIVE THE ILLUSION OF A NARROWER BROW AND CHEEKBONES BY ADDING VOLUME AND
INTEREST TO YOUR JAWLINE.

## makeup

**Eyebrows** Slightly shorten the natural length of
your eyebrows and shape them into a gentle arch.
**Eye shadow** Highlight the center of the eyelid
and create a rounded shape at the outer corners.
**Blush** Apply only to the apples of the cheeks.
**Lipstick** Make your mouth appear wider using
liner, and fill in the color right to the edge.
**Top tip** Lip glosses and sheens are a must.

## hairstyle

Your hairstyle should add volume and interest to
your jawline. A one-length bob that finishes just
below your earlobe and that is turned in or
flipped out is ideal. Pulled-back styles or styles that
add volume around the temples are not for you;
bangs should be light and feathered.

## eyeglasses

The frames should not extend beyond your
temples. Frameless eyeglasses are an excellent
choice, and the arms should be lightweight.

## earrings

Choose large earrings that will draw attention to
your jawline. Dangly styles are great if you have a
long neck.

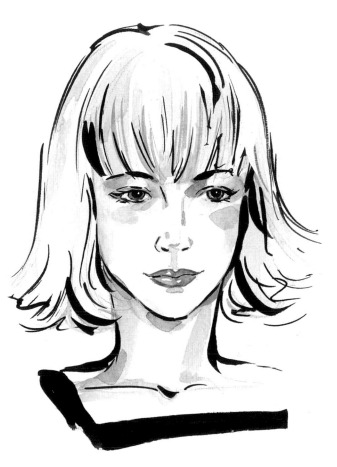

For more advice on applying makeup:
**go to pages 171–179.**

# round

ALTHOUGH THE SOFTNESS OF A ROUND FACE CAN BE ATTRACTIVE, CREATING ANGLES AND VERTICAL LINES THROUGH YOUR CHOICE OF HAIRSTYLE AND CLEVER APPLICATION OF MAKEUP WILL HELP GIVE THE ILLUSION OF A MORE BALANCED FACE SHAPE.

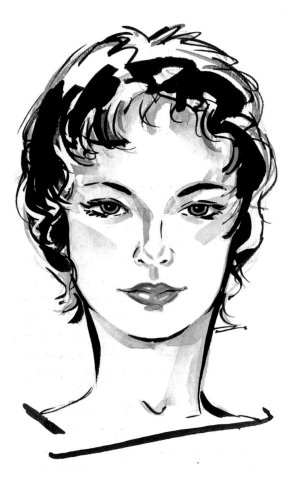

## makeup

**Eyebrows** Keep your eyebrows as straight as possible, and don't let the outer corner droop.
**Eye shadow** Apply colors in diagonal lines that slant up toward the outer corners of your eyes.
**Blush** Apply blush in a straight line along the cheekbones.
**Lipstick** Create a wider, slightly narrower mouth when lining your lips.
**Top tip** Use a highlighter (or shine or gloss) along the top of the cheekbone to create angles.

## hairstyle

Asymmetric parts and bangs are flattering, while a light, feathered style will break up the fullness of the face. Avoid a big, bubbly perm or a rounded bob that frames the face.

## eyeglasses

Frames that are slightly wider than your face will make your face seem smaller. Square or rectangular frames balance a round face, but avoid round shapes and full, frameless lenses.

## earrings

Choose angled or dangly styles (if you have a long neck), but avoid round or hooped earrings.

For more advice on applying makeup: **go to pages 171–179.**

# makeup know-how

YOU DON'T HAVE TO SPEND HOURS IN FRONT OF THE MIRROR EVERY DAY, BUT YOU DESERVE TO LOOK YOUR BEST AT ALL TIMES. AFTER ALL, RESEARCH HAS SHOWN THAT WOMEN WHO WEAR MAKEUP LOOK YOUNGER, EARN MORE, AND GET PROMOTED MORE QUICKLY. THE FOLLOWING ADVICE HAS HELPED THOUSANDS OF WOMEN ACHIEVE A POLISHED AND GROOMED LOOK WITHOUT BEING OVERLY MADE UP.

In addition to giving you a well-groomed, polished appearance, makeup can work magic. By placing lines and colors in the correct places, you can "adjust" the proportions of your face to create a more balanced face shape, giving the illusion of a smaller nose, bigger eyes, or a smaller chin, for example.

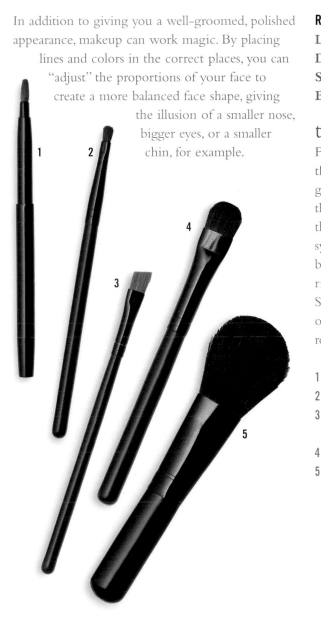

**REMEMBER THESE PRINCIPLES:**

**Light colors** highlight and draw attention
**Dark colors** make things look smaller
**Soft** and **muted colors** minimize
**Bright** and **clear colors** emphasize

## tool kit

For the most successful results, you need to use the correct makeup tools. Treat yourself to some good-quality brushes. Natural bristle brushes are the preferred choice of makeup artists, because they are gentler on the skin and shed less than synthetic brushes. Keep them in good condition by washing them once a week in mild shampoo; rinse well, blot, then stand them upright to dry. Storing your tools in one place—in the bathroom or on a dressing table—will help speed up your routine. Below are the key items you will need.

| | |
|---|---|
| 1 Lip brush | Cosmetic sponge |
| 2 Concealer brush | Powder brush |
| 3 Angled eye shadow brush | Eyelash curlers |
| | Pencil sharpener |
| 4 Blender brush | Cotton pads |
| 5 Blush brush | Cotton swabs (Q-tips) |

# application techniques

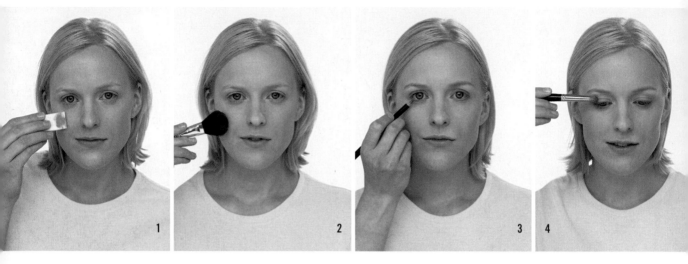

These basic makeup application techniques and tips will help you achieve professional results. You can adapt the steps depending on how long you want to spend on your makeup, and on the occasion. For example, for a day at work you may want nothing more than a light base, such as a tinted moisturizer, and a slick of mascara. For a special night out, though, you may wish to emphasize your eyes more than usual with eyeliner and several shades of eye shadow, or play up your lips. Whatever your routine, whether you wear a little makeup or a lot, always start with a clean and freshly moisturized face.

## STEP 1—FOUNDATION

First of all, use a skintone adjuster to camouflage any blemishes, broken veins or dark circles under the eyes. Most skintone adjusters come in two shades: green to counteract red blemishes; yellow to counteract dark shadows and pink blemishes.

Apply foundation or tinted moisturizer, using either a cosmetic sponge or your fingertips and working on one part of the face at a time. Avoid your eyelids and lips, and do not dot the foundation over your nose, forehead, cheeks, and chin—it will dry as it contacts the air and result in uneven coverage. Finally, apply concealer to hide any visible blemishes.

## STEP 2—POWDER

To set your makeup, apply loose powder to the bony areas of your face with a cotton pad to press the powder in. Use downward strokes with your powder brush to remove excess powder.

## STEP 3—EYELINER

Using an appropriate shade of eye pencil, line the outer third of the lower lid, and the outer two-thirds of the upper lid. Use the pencil from the outer edge of the eye and work inward.

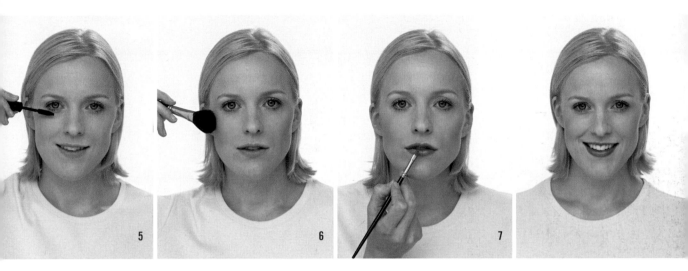

## STEP 4—EYE SHADOW

Apply an eye base evenly all over the eyelids to fix your eye shadow and prevent it from creasing. Following the guidelines for your particular eye shape (page 176), use a blender brush to apply highlighter or a light or neutral shade of eye shadow from the lashes to the eyebrow. Then add a dark, neutral, or accent eye shadow along the lower third of the eyelid and blend. You can use up to four shades of eye shadow if you wish.

## STEP 5—BROWS AND LASHES

Brush your eyebrows against the direction of growth, then brush them back into shape. If necessary, use an eyebrow pencil to lengthen and correct the shape and color (pages 166–170). Curled lashes open up the eye; start close to the roots and work toward the tips, maintaining even pressure. Apply one to two coats of mascara to your top and bottom lashes, concentrating on the tips. Separate the lashes using an eyelash comb before the mascara dries.

## STEP 6—BLUSH

Apply blush along the cheekbones, following the guidelines relating to your face shape (pages 166–170) and building up the color gradually to the desired depth. Powder blush should be applied with a brush, while cream blush, which is more forgiving on older skin, can be applied with a brush or fingertips.

## STEP 7—LIPS

Apply lip base to make your lipstick last longer. Follow the guidelines for your particular lip shape (page 177). Outline your lips with a pencil and fill in for more depth of color. Apply lipstick, blot, then reapply and finish with lip gloss if you wish. If you want to slightly change the shade of your lipstick, try a different color lip pencil.

# evening glamour

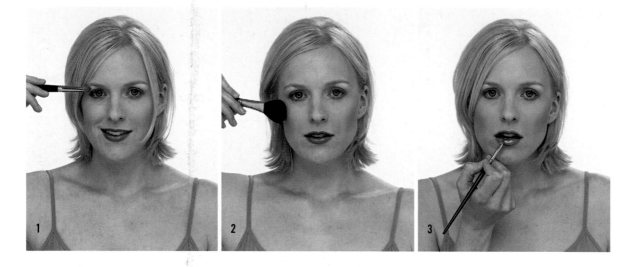

1  2  3

Sometimes, a little magic is needed to transform you at the end of a hectic day. Even if you don't have time to start from scratch, these tips will help take you from daytime beauty to evening belle. Refer to the techniques on the previous pages, but note that your face needs more color in artificial light, so choose stronger shades for eyes and lips. Remove your makeup (leave your eye makeup intact if you don't have much time). Apply moisturizer, then reapply your foundation, concealer, and powder.

## STEP 1—THE EYES

Use a darker shade of eye pencil and a brighter accent eye shadow (or one with a sheen). A dash of gold or silver powder on the center of both eyelids will make your eyes sparkle. Reapply your mascara, emphasizing the outer edges of the eyes to give a wide-eyed expression. Reapply your eyebrow color if necessary.

## STEP 2—THE CHEEKS

Choose a deeper shade of blush from your palette to give your cheeks more color and definition. Apply blush to the apple of your cheek, working upward and outward.

## STEP 3—THE LIPS

Choose either the darkest or brightest lipstick color from your palette. Apply lip base for more staying power, then line and fill in your lips with a toning lip liner. Apply lipstick as before, then add a coat of gloss for extra sheen.

## STEP 4—FINISHING TOUCHES

Using a large powder brush, sweep bronzing powder over the prominent parts of your face (temples, cheekbones, chin, and tip of nose). Stand back from the mirror and look at your face from a distance to check the overall effect. Don't forget a splash of perfume.

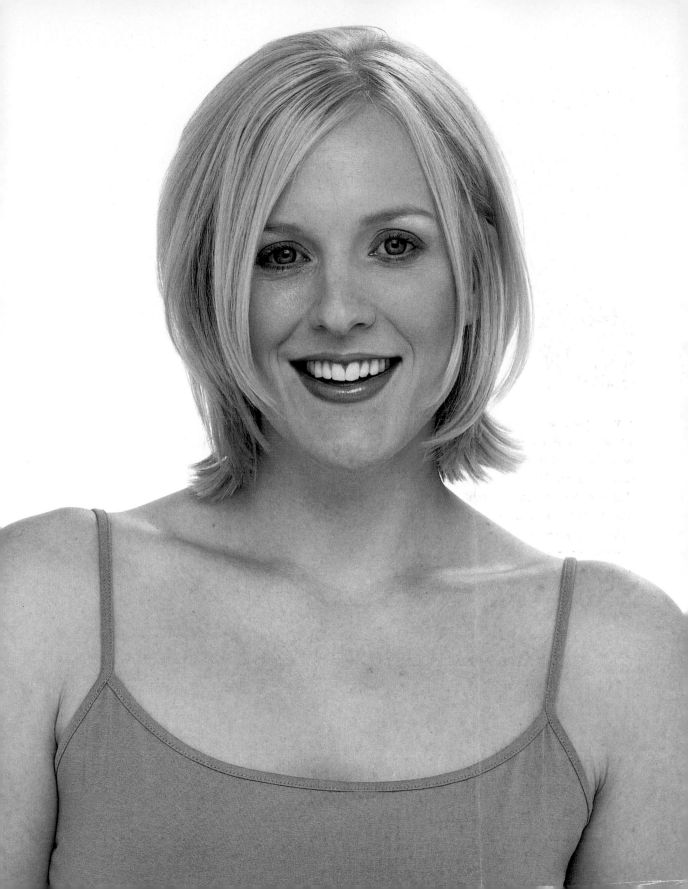

# the eyes have it

EYES COME IN ALL SHAPES AND SIZES—CLOSE-SET, DEEP-SET, SLANTING, AND WITH SMALL OR LARGE LIDS. AS WITH DIFFERENT FACE SHAPES, THERE ARE VARIOUS MAKEUP TRICKS YOU CAN EMPLOY TO BALANCE THE SHAPE OF YOUR EYES AND SHOW THEM OFF TO THEIR BEST ADVANTAGE. THE MOST COMMON PROBLEMS AND SOLUTIONS ARE GIVEN BELOW.

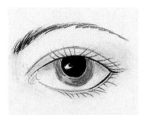 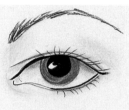 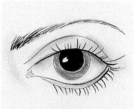 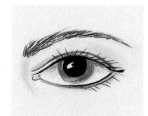

### PROPORTIONED OR ALMOND-SHAPED EYES

- Two-thirds of the eye area is brow and one-third is lid.
- Using a blender brush, apply highlighter from lashes to brow.
- Line the outer two-thirds of the top lid and one-third of the lower lid with pencil.
- Using an angled brush, apply a neutral shade of eye shadow along the orbital bone.
- Apply an accent color to the upper lid, ending in a triangle at the outer corner.
- Finally, apply neutral eye shadow to blend.

### SMALL LIDS, LARGE BROW AREA

- Balance the eye by creating a natural contour on the brow area and light colors on the eyelids.
- With a blender brush, apply matte highlighter from lashes to brow.
- Line two-thirds of the lower lid and one-third of the top lid.
- Use an angled brush to apply a neutral shade of eye shadow in a wide arch over the fleshiest part of the eye.
- Add accent color over eyeliner, keeping the eyelid light.

### PROMINENT LIDS, SMALL BROW AREA

- The sockets may seem deep-set and the brow area narrow. Make the lids less prominent and elongate the eyes.
- Using a blender brush, apply a light or neutral shade to the eye lids and brows.
- Line the bottom lid with a dark pencil and apply a wide line across the top lid, blending upward and outward at the corner.
- Apply a similar color over the entire lid, then blend with a soft or neutral shadow.
- Apply lots of mascara.

### SMALL LIDS, SMALL BROW AREA

- Shape your eyebrows to increase the eye area.
- Apply highlighter over the whole area with a blender brush.
- Line two-thirds of the bottom lid and one-third of the top lid with pencil, extending slightly beyond the outer corner.
- Apply an accent shadow close to the lashes on the top lid, winging up and out at the corner.
- Apply the same color over the pencil on the lower lids. Use a neutral shade to blend.

# the lips have it

THE PERFECT POUT IS THE CROWNING GLORY TO YOUR MAKEUP, BUT IT TAKES A LITTLE WORK TO GET IT JUST RIGHT. WHETHER YOUR MOUTH IS FULL, THIN, WIDE, OR SMALL, MAKE THE MOST OF IT BY FOLLOWING THE GUIDELINES BELOW. REMEMBER, FILLING IN THE LIPS WITH PENCIL GIVES DEFINITION, AND YOU SHOULD ALWAYS BLOT AFTER THE FIRST COAT OF LIPSTICK, THEN REAPPLY.

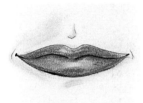 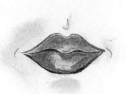 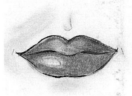 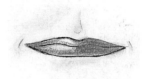

### WIDE MOUTH

- The aim is to make your mouth appear fuller and smaller.
- Apply lip pencil within the inside corner of the mouth.
- Fill in the color, then apply two coats of lipstick.
- Apply gloss only to the center of the lips.

### SMALL MOUTH

- The aim is to give the illusion of a wider and fuller mouth.
- Apply lip pencil to extend the outer edges of the mouth and fill in the color.
- Use a lip brush to apply your lipstick, making sure you cover all of the new shape you have created.
- Apply gloss all over the lips.

### FULL LIPS

- The darkest shades in your palette work best. Avoid high-sheen and frosted formulations, which will make your lips look bigger.
- Apply lip pencil within the natural lip line and fill in for extra definition.
- Apply two coats of lipstick, blotting after the first coat.

### THIN LIPS

- The lightest lipstick shades in your palette work best.
- Apply lip pencil just beyond the natural lip line and fill in the color for definition.
- Using a lip brush, apply a coat of lipstick, blot, and reapply.
- Use a sheer lipstick or gloss to highlight the center of the lower lip.

## UNBALANCED LIPS

If one lip is fuller than the other, balance them using one light and one dark shade. On the fuller lip, apply lip pencil within the natural line of the lip; on the thinner lip, apply pencil beyond the natural line. Apply a darker lipstick to the fuller lip and a lighter shade to the thinner lip.

# changing faces

NOTHING DATES A WOMAN AS MUCH AS WEARING THE SAME MAKEUP AT 50 AS SHE DID WHEN SHE WAS 25—YOUR STYLE OF MAKEUP AND THE WAY YOU APPLY IT SHOULD CHANGE AS YOU MATURE. A GOOD SKINCARE REGIME AND A HEALTHY LIFESTYLE, ALONG WITH THE RIGHT CLOTHES, COLORS, AND STYLE, ARE ESSENTIAL FOR LOOKING GOOD AND FEELING CONFIDENT. HERE ARE A FEW WINNING TIPS TO HELP YOU EVOLVE YOUR LOOK.

## when you are 30–40

- You should have established a good skincare routine: cleansing, toning, and moisturizing every day; exfoliating and applying a treatment mask appropriate to your skin type—dry, oily, sensitive, or normal—once a week.
- Ensure that you are using high-factor sunblocks all year round to protect your skin from harmful UVB rays and aging UVA rays.

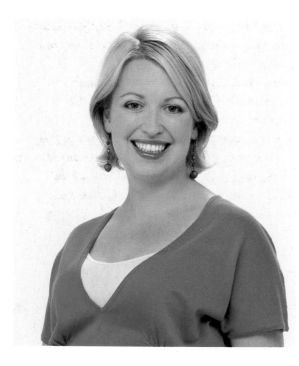

*A good skincare regime and a healthy lifestyle will keep you looking and feeling good*

- Learn to recognize good-quality cosmetic products that offer the most benefits.
- Wear makeup every day to protect your skin.
- You are no longer a teenager, so makeup with glitter and sparkle should only be worn for parties, and even then in moderation.
- High-fashion makeup looks are for runway models only.
- Make regular appointments with a hygienist to ensure that you have a dazzling smile.

## when you are 40–50

- Keep positive when the first gray hairs and lines start to appear.
- Throw away frosted eye shadows, glossy lipsticks, and colored mascaras. Don't overdo the fake tan, and avoid orangey shades.
- Feed and nourish your skin regularly.
- Stick to a simple makeup routine, applying a minimum of base (foundation or tinted moisturizer and concealer as necessary), blush, mascara, and lipstick.

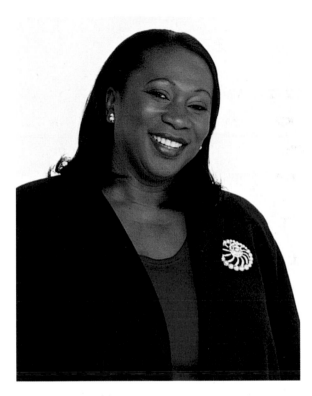

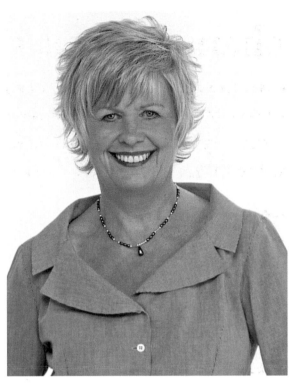

- Don't be afraid to use a little powder to create a more groomed look, but be careful not to apply too much, and make sure you blend it well, because it can collect in and draw attention to fine lines.
- Use blushs and bronzers to emphasize facial bone structure and add definition to your face, particularly if you're carrying a little extra weight here.

## when you are 50 +

- Indulge yourself with the occasional pampering treat at a spa or beauty salon.
- A skincare regime is a must. Now is the time to use products that have been specially formulated for mature skins.
- Keep abreast of the latest beauty technology so that you can benefit from new products.

- Don't forget the rest of your body. Use a skin-firming moisturizer morning and night, and always after bathing.
- Pay special attention to your décolletage—smooth face cream downward and body cream upward.
- Your beauty routine will now include paying more attention to your eyebrows. Besides shaping, they may need to have a little color added.
- Less is more when it comes to makeup.
- An eye base is now essential—it will prevent your lids from looking creased when wearing eye shadow.
- A lip base will help prevent lipstick from bleeding and avoid a "buttonhole" lip.
- Use powder on the bony parts of your face only, and avoid the soft, fleshy areas, such as eyelids and the area just below the eyes.

# underwear

OVERDECORATED UNDERWEAR WILL SHOW THROUGH CLOSE-FITTING GARMENTS. UNDERWEAR SHOULD COORDINATE WITH THE COLORS OF YOUR OUTER GARMENTS, AND SHOULD NOT BE SEEN UNLESS YOU'RE MAKING A FASHION STATEMENT.

## bras

A bra is an important investment—it provides essential support for your breasts and creates the foundation for your outfit.

- Buy bras for different outfits and occasions: seamless, strapless, sports, and so on.
- Get measured professionally once a year and try on a range of styles from different brands—some cuts will fit you better than others.
- The back of your bra should sit in the middle of your back.
- Your breasts should not hang over the cups.
- If you have heavy breasts, a bra with nonstretch straps will be more supportive.
- If you have a fleshy back, three hooks are better than two.
- Fasten a new bra on the widest hooks and move inward as the bra stretches with wear.

## panties

There is no excuse for visible panty lines (VPLs); with so much choice available, you should be able to find a cut and fit that are right for you.

- Buy bigger-sized panties than you think you will need. This will eliminate visible panty lines by ensuring that the elastic doesn't cut into your flesh. Panties are also notorious for shrinking in the wash.
- If you need tummy control, make sure the fit is good and that your flesh doesn't roll over the top when you sit down.

## pantyhose

A woman used not to be considered properly dressed unless she wore pantyhose, whatever the weather. Nowadays, unless you work in a formal environment or are attending a formal event, it is usually acceptable to go without pantyhose in the summer, as long as your legs are hair- and blemish-free. However, always wear pantyhose with a suit.

- Natural-colored pantyhose are suitable for most occasions.
- To elongate the legs, wear pantyhose that are the same color as your skirt or shoes.
- Balance the denier of your pantyhose with the fabric weight of your skirt or pants. In the summer, with a lightweight fabric, seven to ten denier is ideal. In the winter, with corduroy or tweed, you may consider opaques (30+ denier).
- Textured pantyhose will give your outfit a fun twist, but they can add volume to the leg.

# accessories

SHOES AND BOOTS WILL UPDATE YOUR LOOK EASILY, SO YOU SHOULD INVEST IN AT LEAST ONE NEW PAIR
EVERY SEASON. BAGS AND HATS ARE ALSO KEY ITEMS IN CREATING YOUR LOOK AND ARE A GOOD WAY TO
REINFORCE YOUR STYLE PERSONALITY. BELTS ARE USEFUL FOR BALANCING YOUR PROPORTIONS, BUT THE
STYLE YOU CHOOSE AND HOW YOU WEAR IT WILL DEPEND ON YOUR BODY SHAPE. SCARVES ARE A GREAT WAY
TO INTRODUCE YOUR COLORS.

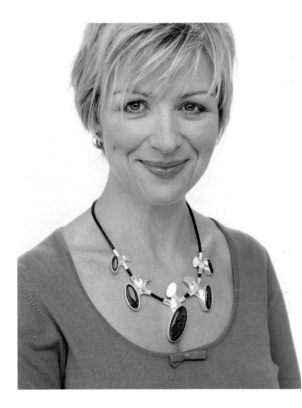

*Accessories are the easiest way to introduce color into your wardrobe*

## jewelry

If making a statement, just wear one piece so that you don't overpower your look; otherwise your jewelry should balance with your scale.

## hats

Hats date quickly and won't necessarily have much longevity in your wardrobe. However, they can turn a plain outfit into something special.

- Brims should not extend beyond your shoulders.
- Grand-scale women should avoid pillbox hats, which will look out of proportion.
- Petite women should not be tempted by large, wide-brimmed hats (picture hats).
- Complement your face with your hat shape. Rounded crowns, and brims in loosely woven straw or soft fabrics, suit round faces.
- Square or rectangular faces will look good in flat crowns and straight brims.
- A downward-sloping brim doesn't work with a short neck, and can emphasize jowls; a brim with an upward tilt will help lift the face.
- A completely coordinated outfit with matching hat looks contrived; a complementary or contrasting color adds interest to an outfit.
- Dark colors cast a shadow over your face.

## scarves

Even if you don't own many clothes in your colors, a scarf is a great way to experiment and instantly gives you the right shade near your face.

- Petite women should avoid oversized scarves, such as full-size pashminas, as these can swamp your appearance.
- Skinny scarves will look out of proportion on grand-scale women.
- Do not tie scarves under your chin if you have a short neck.
- A long, thin scarf draped around your neck will make your body appear taller and slimmer.

## belts

Belts are great fashion accessories that can update your look. Worn cleverly, belts can also help balance the proportions of your upper and lower body and define the waist.

- You need a waist to wear a belt, so they are not ideal for Lean Columns, Rectangles, or Round body shapes.
- Narrow and lightweight belts are best on petite to average women.
- Wide, statement belts are best on average to grand-scale women.
- Belts must work with the rest of your look.

## bags

Besides carrying belongings, your handbag makes a style statement, and the bag you choose will be dictated by your style personality: *go to pages 146–161*. Like shoes, a bag can make or break your look, so here are some key pointers to help you make a choice:

- Different occasions call for different styles and sizes of handbag, so try to build up a collection that is appropriate for various occasions and outfits. Don't take a floral straw bag to a business meeting, nor a formal leather handbag to a dinner dance.
- Your bag needs to be in balance with your overall scale: a large bag will overwhelm a petite person, while a tiny bag will look lost on a grand-scale woman.
- The shape of your bag needs to follow the line of your body.
- Rectangles, Lean Columns, and Inverted Triangles need structured bags to reflect the lines and angles of their bodies.

- Softer, unstructured bags work best for those with a Full Hourglass or Round shape.
- Triangles should avoid bags that hang at hip level, as they will add width to the widest area.
- Before you buy a handbag, look at yourself carrying it to make sure it looks right for you.

## footwear

Like all your accessories, the type of shoes or boots you wear can kill your look, so make sure they are appropriate for your outfit. Here are some guidelines for buying shoes and boots:

- The heel height you choose will often be determined by your comfort level, but a high or a narrow heel always adds length to the leg.
- If you are wearing a short skirt, a lower heel will make your legs look longer.
- Low-fronted shoes give the illusion of longer legs and narrower ankles; closed shoes shorten the length of the feet and legs.
- When choosing shoes with straps, bear in mind that low-cut t-straps work for most people, while ankle straps will only look good on those with long legs and slim ankles.
- When buying boots, check that the boot— whether ankle, calf-height, or full-length—stops at a narrow point on your legs.
- Sandals are ideal for vacations and hot weather, but your feet must be in immaculate condition. They should never be worn with business suits.
- Ballet flats are wonderful for anyone with average to long legs and thin ankles. Satin, velvet, or beaded flats are good choices for evening, teamed with long skirts or pants.

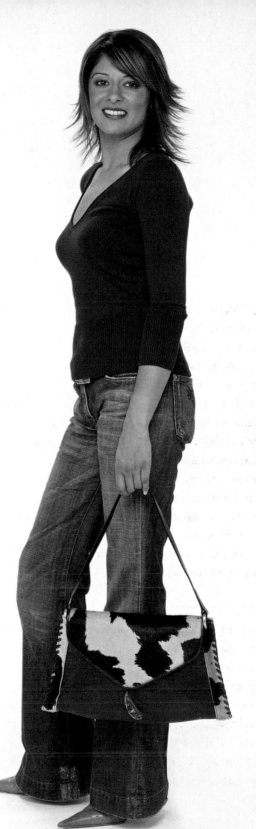

# looking beautiful with a bump

BEING PREGNANT WILL GIVE MOST WOMEN SOME NEW CHALLENGES IN THE WARDROBE DEPARTMENT. YOUR BODY SHAPE AND WEIGHT WILL CHANGE OVER THE MONTHS, AND THERE WILL BE EMOTIONAL HIGHS AND LOWS DUE TO ALL THE HORMONE CHANGES TAKING PLACE. TO FEEL CONFIDENT DURING THIS EXCITING TIME, A LITTLE THOUGHT ABOUT WHAT YOU CHOOSE TO WEAR WILL MAKE THIS A MORE PLEASURABLE EXPERIENCE.

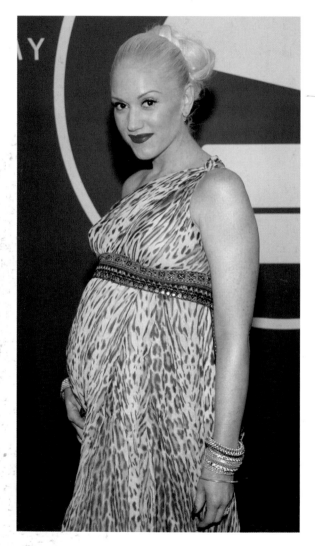

## the months ahead

- During your pregnancy, your proportions will not change, although your waist definition will go. So the general rules on proportions will remain the same: *go to pages 136–138*.
- To ensure that pregnancy doesn't take a toll on your bust, it is important to be fitted regularly over the coming months, as your bust size will definitely increase.
- There will be times when your energy levels sink; color will give you the boost you need, and will help you look healthier and fitter: *go to pages 34–105*.

## early days

Your bust starts enlarging and your waist begins to thicken, but you can fit into your "normal" clothes.

- Check out your closet for shirts, cardigans, empire-style dresses, and tops that will accommodate these changes.
- Pants and skirts can be left slightly undone, as long as this doesn't affect the way they hang.
- Shorter dresses and tunics look great over leggings, or over jeans and pants where you may not be able to fasten the waist.
- As much as you may be tempted to wear your partner's baggy tracksuit bottoms, this is to be avoided at all costs!

# blooming days

You will now start telling the world about your forthcoming event. However, this doesn't mean you have to wear a tent! You need to purchase a few key pieces that will take you through the following months and that you can accessorize for fun and color. If you're buying specially designed maternity clothes, stick to your "normal" size. Small and petite women may find that they have to go one or two sizes larger and shorten the garments.

## PANTS

Your first stop should be to find the best-fitting pants and/or jeans that will accommodate your expanding bump.

## DRESSES

Dresses will be a longer-lasting option than a skirt. Wrap and empire styles are perfect, and fabric with some stretch will gently skim your bump.

## TOPS

How you show off your bump is very much a personal choice. Some women like a tight-fitting look that shows off their natural shape plus bump; others will feel more comfortable in a looser, more fluid garment that discreetly shows their increasing bump.

## SHOES

Your high heels and favorite fashion shoes will need a rest until the baby is born, since the extra weight you will be carrying may make your feet wider and you may wobble on those elegant heels. You can still remain fashionable wearing some well-constructed flats or wedge shoes. Ballet flats are pretty but do not give you the support you need—only wear them occasionally. Do get measured properly to guarantee good support.

## ACCESSORIES

Your "normal" accessories will still work and enhance your look. If you miss your shopping trips, a new pair of earrings or a new handbag will still give you the boost you need. Remember to balance the proportion of your bump with the size of your bag! Thinking ahead, you will need a larger bag for all the baby paraphernalia—and that's a wonderful excuse for a new bag.

# nearly there

Pamper yourself in these later weeks—there won't be time once the baby arrives.

You can still look glamorous and feminine, and don't forsake prettiness for practicality. Have a mani-pedi (a manicure and pedicure at the same time), keep up your skincare and makeup routine, and discuss with your hairdresser a low-maintenance hairstyle for the months to come.

Rings can get tight in the last few weeks, and you may want to store them until you can slip them back on again—buy some fun costume jewelry instead.

# glamming up

IT'S SO EXCITING TO GET AN INVITATION TO A SPECIAL OCCASION, WHETHER IT'S A WEDDING, A CHRISTMAS PARTY, A FAMILY CELEBRATION, OR A SPECIAL NIGHT OUT WITH YOUR FAVORITE DATE. CHOOSING AN OUTFIT THAT IS CURRENT, BUT NOT HIGH FASHION, WILL ENSURE THE LONGEVITY OF THE CLOTHES—THAT ASYMMETRIC SHOULDER LINE WILL LOOK OUT OF PLACE A YEAR FROM NOW. A SIMPLE DRESS WITH THE RIGHT ACCESSORIES WILL BE DATELESS.

Glamming up will mean different things to different women. This is where understanding your style personality will come into its own: *go to pages 144–161*. Some of you may just want to get the investment jewelry out, while others will rush down to the mall and buy the latest trends.

## CREATIVE

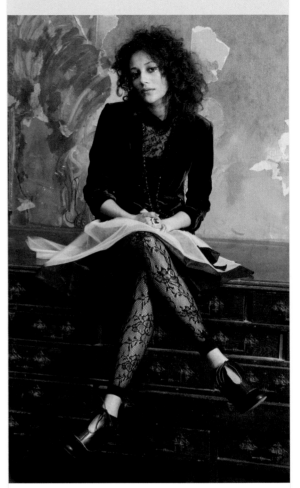

You will have a ball dreaming up something different to wear. Vintage clothes will be a great choice. Try something lacy, and don't forget the antique jewelry and perhaps a beaded bag. In colder weather, go for velvets and velours, and even fake fur.

For more Creative style ideas: **go to pages 150–151**.

## DRESSING FOR THE OCCASION
Make sure that you wear what is appropriate for the event. You do not want to outdo the hostess or be the only guest who has not made an effort. To help you pull the look together, we suggest you find out about:
- The venue: inside or out
- The event: formal or informal
- The time: day or evening

## DRAMATIC

You will definitely want a completely new outfit, but before you rush out, go through your closet and see what is lurking there. Maybe just a new pair of colorful shoes or a new top will give you the wow factor.

For more Dramatic style ideas: **go to pages 152–153**.

## ROMANTIC

You are in your element. You are bound to have something pretty already in your closet, but make sure it is appropriate for the event. If you'll be standing for a long time, you may have to sacrifice the killer heels for a more comfortable pair. Don't forget to book all your pampering treatments ahead of time so that you will really feel glamorous on the day.

For more Romantic style ideas: **go to pages 154–155**.

## CLASSIC

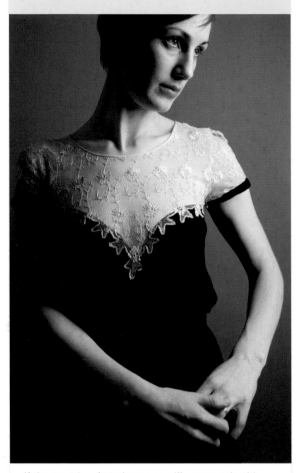

## NATURAL

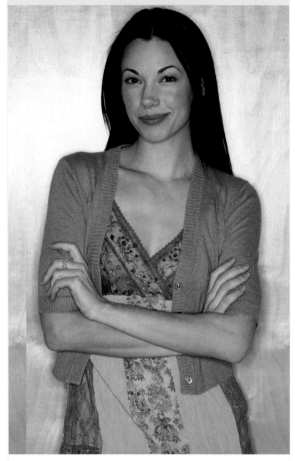

If the event is a formal one, you will wear a suit with coordinated accessories; you may find a less formal event a little more challenging. A dress with a complementary (not matching) pashmina, shrug, or cardigan will be a good alternative. Don't forget to add a little sparkle somewhere, even if it is costume jewelry. Forget the pumps and go for heeled sandals or open-toe wedges.

For more Classic style ideas: **go to pages 156–157**.

This is your least-favorite scenario, so keep it simple and comfortable. Go for a pantsuit for the formal occasion or a long skirt or pants for a more relaxed do. Don't forget to follow the makeup application tips in Chapter 6 for a groomed and polished look: **go to pages 164–177**. Don't feel shy about adding some jewelry; a simple strand of beads looks pretty without being fussy. Your best handbag choice will be one with a long strap.

For more Natural style ideas: **go to pages 158–159**.

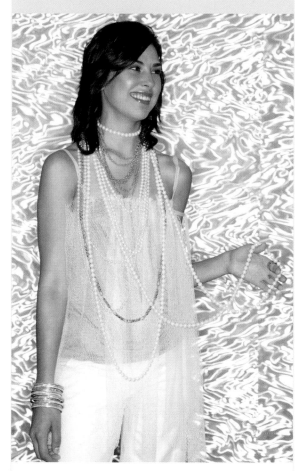

**CITY CHIC**

Your clothes style will remain the same, but the fabrics will be more luxurious: think silks and satins. Add color to your usual neutrals with a scarf or shawl, some stunning jewelry, a dressy handbag, and a fun pair of shoes.

For more City Chic style ideas: **go to pages 160–161**

## finishing touches

Now is the perfect time to indulge in a little pampering and glam up with your hairstyle and makeup.

There is nothing like a good haircut, color and a blow-dry to make you feel like a million dollars. You may even consider adding some sparkling clips or detailed headbands to your finished hairstyle.

Allow plenty of time to apply your makeup and maybe go for a more vibrant or darker lipstick than you would usually wear. A dusting of shimmer anywhere on the face is flattering and glamorous, and a light spray of perfume will complete your outfit.

## underwear

Often your chosen outfit does not work with your normal, everyday lingerie. Thin straps, low backs, and strapless dresses call for special underwear that will still give you the right support and shape, but without unsightly straps showing— there is nothing more embarrassing than, halfway through an event, your bra strap appearing or, worse still, your strapless top beginning to slip.

# perfect packing

MOST WOMEN RETURN FROM THEIR VACATION WITH A SUITCASE OF CLOTHES THEY HAVEN'T WORN. WITH AIRLINES TODAY CHARGING MORE AND MORE FOR CHECKED BAGGAGE, LEARNING TO PACK LIGHT IS THE ORDER OF THE DAY, AND WITH HAND LUGGAGE ONLY, THINK OF THE EXTRA TIME YOU'LL SAVE WHEN YOU ARRIVE AT YOUR DESTINATION.

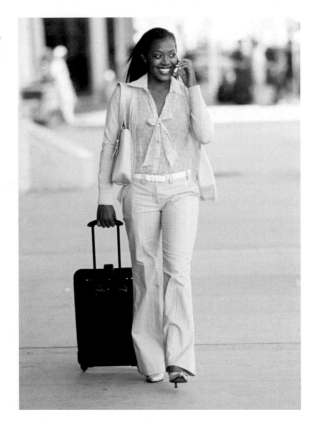

## packing rules

- Pack as few clothes as possible
- Wear your heavier shoes/boots/coat
- Decant your toiletries into travel-sized plastic bottles
- Streamline your makeup bag—you don't need 10 lipsticks and eye shadows
- Wear your valuable jewelry and keep the costume jewelry light
- One perfume only
- Don't go overboard with underwear—it can be washed overnight
- Make sure your traveling handbag is large enough to carry your documents and essentials, and put a pouch inside it that will double as your evening bag.

## your traveling wardrobe

List every day of your trip, and for each day write down what you might be doing (lunch, sightseeing, sporting activity, or just relaxing). For each of these, make a note of what you are likely to wear. This will demonstrate that indeed you can wear the same pair of pants twice, and therefore how little you need to pack.

- Following your list, lay all the clothes out on the bed, and see how they co-ordinate with each other. There is no point in taking the little red sparkly top 'just in case' if you do not pack something to go with it.
- Keep the colors you take to a minimum. Your pants and jacket should be in neutral shades, which will work with everything else.
- If you have forgotten something, have fun and buy it locally! You need to leave some space in your suitcase for anything you may want to bring back.

Opposite are some basic packing guidelines to make your planning easier.

Bon voyage!

## THE CITY BREAK (3 DAYS/2 NIGHTS)

- 1 waterproof jacket/coat
- 1 versatile, neutral jacket that you can glam up
- 1 pair of pants
- 1 pair of jeans
- 1 dress
- 1 skirt
- 1 twinset (sweater + cardigan)
- 1 shirt/blouse
- 1 t-shirt
- 1 pashmina
- 1 pair of loafers/comfortable shoes
- 1 pair of heels
- underwear for 3 days + 1 spare (in case of delay)

| DAY | DAYTIME | EVENING |
|---|---|---|
| 1 TRAVEL | Jacket, pants, sweater (from twinset), loafers | Jacket, dress, heels |
| 2 | Jeans, t-shirt, waterproof/jacket, loafers | Skirt, blouse, heels, pashmina |
| 3 | Pants, twinset, loafers | Dress, cardigan (from twinset), heels |
| TRAVEL HOME | Jeans, blouse, jacket, loafers | |

## THE ONE-WEEK BEACH VACATION

- 1 pair of jeans
- 1 pair of cropped pants
- 1 pair of shorts
- 2 dresses
- 1 skirt
- 1 caftan
- 1 dressy t-shirt
- 3 t-shirts
- 1 cotton twinset (strappy top + cardigan)
- 1 pair of sneaker-style shoes
- 1 pair of pretty sandals or flip-flops
- 1 pair of heels
- 1 pair of ballet pumps
- 1 pashmina
- 3 swimsuits/bikinis
- 1 hat
- underwear for 4 days (do a wash every other day)
- your travel bag will double as a beach bag!

| DAY | AM/PM | EVENING |
|---|---|---|
| 1 TRAVEL | Jeans, twinset, sneaker-style shoes | Cropped pants, dressy t-shirt, pretty sandals |
| 2 BEACH | Shorts, t-shirt 1, sandals/flip-flops | Dress 1, heels, pashmina |
| 3 POOL | Caftan, sandals/flip-flops | Skirt, strappy top, ballet pumps |
| 4 BEACH | Shorts, t-shirt 2, sandals/flip-flops | Dress 2, heels |
| 5 SIGHTSEEING | Cropped pants, t-shirt 1, sneaker-style shoes | Skirt, dressy t-shirt, ballet pumps |
| 6 BEACH | Shorts, t-shirt 3, sandals/flip-flops | Dress 1, heels |
| 7 POOL | Caftan, sandals | Dress 2 or new dress bought locally, heels |
| TRAVEL HOME | Jeans, t-shirt 2, cardigan (from twinset) | |

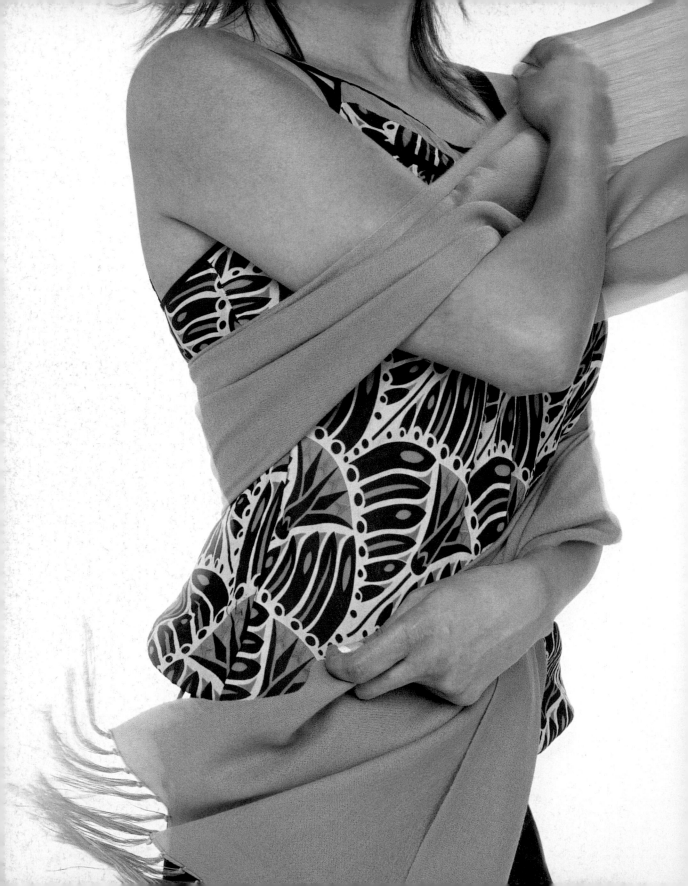

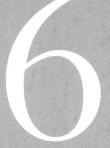

# making your
# closet work

# organizing your closet

NOW THAT YOU'VE ESTABLISHED YOUR COLORS, STYLE PERSONALITY, AND BODY SHAPE, AND SEEN HOW TO PULL A LOOK TOGETHER, YOU HAVE TO MAKE IT ALL WORK FOR YOU. START AT THE PLACE WHERE YOU KEEP MOST OF YOUR CLOTHES: YOUR CLOSET.

## closet inventory

The best way to check out what you have, what works, and what doesn't work in your closet is to go through each item of clothing piece by piece. Allow yourself at least a day to do this.

**YOU WILL END UP WITH THREE PILES:**

**Pile 1** Clothes you will keep
**Pile 2** Clothes you might keep
**Pile 3** Clothes that must go

**HOW YOU DECIDE**

- Is it the right color? If the answer is yes, then ask yourself if it is the right style. If it is, it goes in pile 1.
- If it's the right color but the wrong style, can it be altered or worn differently to make it work? If it can, it goes in pile 2.
- Is it the right style but the wrong color? Can you wear it with a complementary color from your palette? Do you have a scarf in a color that will make it work? If yes, it goes in pile 2.
- If it's the wrong color and the wrong style, it goes in pile 3.
- If it's not your current size and you haven't worn it for a year, it goes in pile 3.

## PILE 1—CLOTHES FOR KEEPS

- Organize garments by categories: coats, jackets, suits, skirts, pants, dresses, blouses, and shirts. Grouping by color within these categories will give you ideas for combining clothes.
- Button up jackets and coats, and pull up zippers, so that garments hang straight before you put them in the closet, all facing the same way.
- Don't put anything back in the closet unless it's clean.
- Don't overcrowd your closet.

## PILE 2—IS IT WORTH KEEPING?

- Check every piece against what you have in your closet to see whether it is worth keeping. You might find that a jacket in the wrong color, for example, can be made to work for you if worn with a top that you've decided to keep.
- Shortening the hem will salvage a skirt that's too long.
- Changing the buttons on a jacket will give it a new lease on life.

## PILE 3—DISPOSE OF CLOTHES AS YOU SEE FIT

- Give them to a friend.
- Sell expensive items and those that are still current and of good quality.
- Donate them to a thrift store.

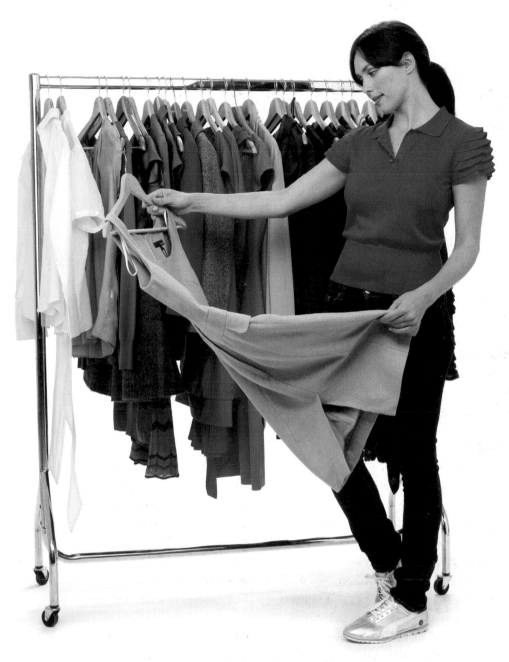

# finishing touches

Before you put everything back in your closet, vacuum and dust it, and perhaps place some moth-repellent products at the bottom. To preserve the shape of your clothes, you will need the correct hangers.

- Sturdy wooden hangers for jackets and coats.
- Wooden hangers with clips for skirts and pants.
- Padded hangers for lightweight and delicate, luxury fabrics.
- Basic plastic hangers for blouses, shirts, and lightweight summer dresses.

# how to shop

INEVITABLY, IN THE COURSE OF ORGANIZING YOUR CLOSET, YOU WILL DISPOSE OF ITEMS THAT NEED TO BE REPLACED IN COLORS AND STYLES THAT SUIT YOU. TO HELP YOU IN THIS NEXT PHASE, MAKE A LIST OF WHAT YOU NEED TO COMPLETE YOUR CLOSET.

## investment buys

It's not the cost of an investment buy that matters, it's how often you wear it. A bargain garment that you wear only once is a costly purchase compared with an expensive item that you wear a hundred times. Investment pieces will vary according to your lifestyle and personality, but they will consist of **overcoats**, **jackets**, **skirts, dresses,** and **pants**.

## fashion buys

These are the items that you buy every year to keep your core closet updated and that are fun to wear. They can be anything from a current color or the latest style in tops or dresses.

## it's the fit that counts

- Sizes will vary depending on where you shop and the cut of the item.
- The looser the fit, the slimmer you look—and you'll undoubtedly feel more comfortable.

*Investment pieces should form the core of your closet*

## achieving an elegantly loose fit

- You should be able to fit a finger underneath a waistband.
- Side seams should hang straight, with no horizontal creases.
- Zippers should lie flat.
- Allow some give in the sleeve around the upper arm.
- Skirts and pants should hang straight from the buttocks and not curve under.
- Sleeves on jackets and coats should finish at the wrist.
- Pockets shouldn't gape.
- There should be no pulling around the bust on jackets, blouses, or dresses.

## recognizing quality

- Seams should lie flat and not pull or wrinkle.
- Hemlines should be flat and even.
- Linings or facings must lie flat and not show.
- An expensive price tag doesn't always mean a quality finish.
- Buttonholes should not have loose threads.

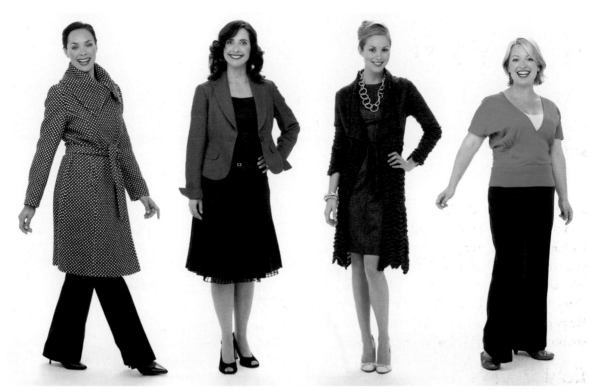

OVERCOATS          JACKETS          SKIRTS/DRESSES          PANTS

## shopping tips

- Make a list, but don't be overambitious about how much you can achieve in one trip.
- Wear appropriate underwear.
- Take along the shoes you'll be wearing with the garment you're buying.
- Look first for the right color: *go to pages 34–109*; then make sure the style suits your body shape, proportions, and scale: *go to pages 112–143*; and, finally, your style personality: *go to pages 146–161*.
- Take only three or four pieces at a time into the fitting room.
- Make sure the item fits and feels comfortable.
- Do you like yourself in it?
- If it's over your budget, is it really worth it?
- Beware of the overenthusiastic salesclerk.

## keeping it looking good

- Clothes that crease easily, such as linens, need laundering after each wearing; tailored suits need to be hung up in order for them to air.
- Shoes absorb moisture when they're worn, which needs to evaporate before you wear them again.
- Keep dry-cleaning to a minimum—the fluids will damage and weaken the fibers.
- Repair any damage to your clothes (loose hems, missing buttons, or snags) immediately.
- Clean shoes regularly, and use shoe trees.

# formal capsule

YOU DON'T NEED A CLOSET FULL OF CLOTHES TO BE WELL DRESSED FOR WORK AND FORMAL OCCASIONS. BY DEVELOPING A "CAPSULE" CLOSET OF BASIC PIECES THAT YOU CAN MIX AND MATCH, YOU CAN BE CONFIDENT OF LOOKING YOUR BEST, WHATEVER THE OCCASION.

## main closet

**SUITS/JACKETS, SKIRTS, AND PANTS** Four suits in complementary neutral colors, or a combination of four jackets and four skirts or pairs of pants.

**TOPS** Six to eight tops, shirts, or knitwear items in your colors. Tops are a good way of introducing color to your closet—if you choose white for the majority of your tops, you'll look the same every day.

**DRESSES** You can wear dresses instead of skirts and tops.

**OVERCOAT** One coat or raincoat that will fit over your suit.

## accessories

**SHOES** Three pairs of formal shoes that fit with current trends and are appropriate for the season.

**BAGS** Two quality handbags, in appropriate colors. If you're using them for work, make sure they're large enough to hold documents and folders. Avoid struggling with laptops and briefcases—a small suitcase on wheels may be the answer.

## dressing tips

- To appear friendly and approachable, you need to wear colors of medium depth. Black and other dark shades represent authority, while red makes you appear assertive: *go to pages 28–31*.
- To look efficient, your grooming has to be impeccable. If your hair is unwashed, you will give the impression of not caring about yourself. If you haven't applied any makeup, other people may think that you're not in control of your time management.
- Complete your formal look from head to toe: a tailored suit calls for toned-down accessories, and pantyhose are essential, whatever the time of year.
- Check your look in a mirror before you leave for the office or event: pretend to pick something off the floor and look at what you see—watch out for that cleavage. Sit down, and see how far your skirt rides up.
- Showing too much skin isn't appropriate in a business or formal environment. Exceptionally long nails are also unsuitable.

For advice on what styles will flatter your body shape the most: *go to pages 112–143*;
for a selection of key pieces in different styles: *go to pages 130–135*.

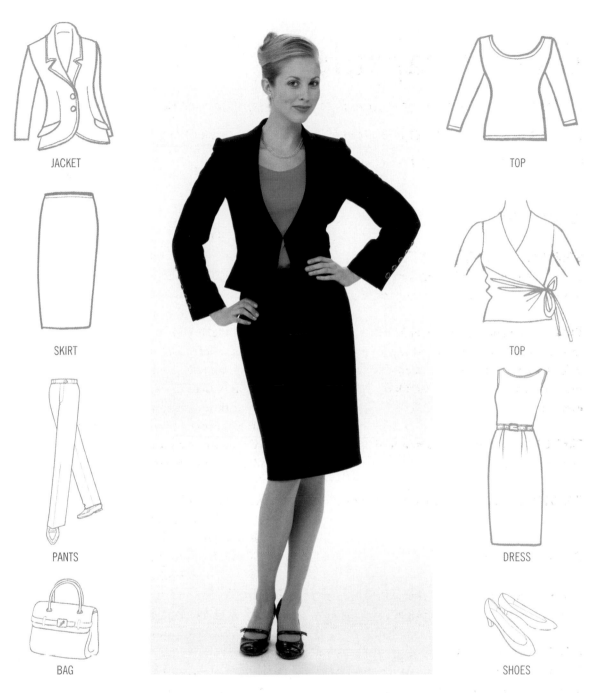

JACKET

TOP

SKIRT

TOP

PANTS

DRESS

BAG

SHOES

*Your business look needs to reflect the core values
of the industry in which you work*

# casual capsule

AS WITH YOUR FORMAL WEAR (PAGES 198–199), A "CAPSULE" CLOSET OF BASIC CASUAL PIECES THAT YOU CAN MIX AND MATCH WILL ALLOW YOU TO PUT TOGETHER A NUMBER OF DIFFERENT OUTFITS WITHOUT BREAKING THE BANK. REMEMBER, THOUGH, THAT A CASUAL LOOK DOESN'T MEAN THAT YOU DON'T NEED TO CARE ABOUT YOUR APPEARANCE.

## main closet

**JACKETS OR CARDIGANS** Four jackets or cardigans, or maybe one jacket, two cardigans, and one fleece.

**SKIRTS, PANTS OR JEANS** Six of these—a combination of whichever you prefer and feel most comfortable in.

**TOPS** Eight tops, from t-shirts to sweaters.

**DRESSES** These can be substituted for the skirt and top options.

## accessories

**SHOES** Four pairs of shoes, boots, or sneakers.

**BAGS** Two handbags that complement your particular lifestyle.

## dressing tips

- Maintain the quality and fit of your clothing.
- Loose-fitting clothing, provided it suits your body shape, is perfect for a smart casual look, but make sure that the fabric doesn't cling to your body.
- Coordinating separates in soft, textured fabrics can replace formal jackets, skirts, and pants.
- Give your dresses a different look by teaming them with either a wrap or a cardigan.
- Think about separating your formal suits and wearing the jackets with a casual skirt, pair of slacks, or dress.
- Dirty, faded, damaged or unkempt clothing isn't acceptable at any time.

For advice on what styles will flatter your body shape the most: *go to pages 112–143*; for a selection of key pieces in different styles: *go to pages 130–135*.

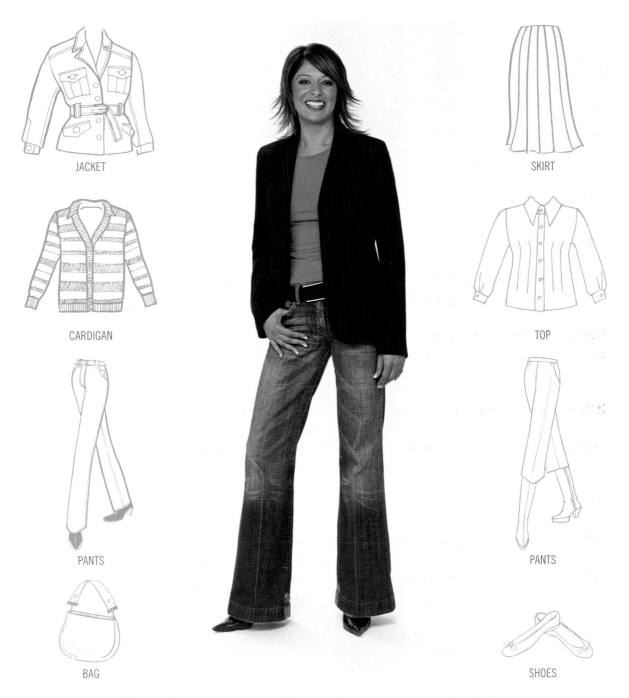

JACKET

CARDIGAN

PANTS

BAG

SKIRT

TOP

PANTS

SHOES

*When dressing casually, make sure you don't let
your grooming standards slip*

# planning for the future

BY MATCHING YOUR LIFESTYLE TO YOUR CLOSET, YOU'LL END UP WITH MORE CLOTHES THAT YOU ACTUALLY WEAR. CREATE TWO PIE CHARTS, ONE REFLECTING YOUR DAILY ACTIVITIES, THE OTHER THE CONTENTS OF YOUR CLOSET. IF THEY DON'T MATCH UP, TAKE ACTION TO MAKE YOUR CLOTHES SUIT YOUR LIFESTYLE WITH THE HELP OF THE CHECKLIST OPPOSITE.

## pie charts

Draw two pie charts. Divide the first chart into sections to reflect the amount of time you spend each day doing the following activities:

**Working**
**At home/taking care of children**
**Social/entertainment**
**Leisure/hobbies**
**Errands**

Divide the second pie chart into sections to reflect what your closet holds, using the same headings.

If you spend 50 percent of your time in the office, then 50 percent of your closet should be represented by your work clothes. Likewise, if you spend only 5 percent of your time socializing, only 5 percent of your closet should be for social occasions, and so on.

If the charts don't match, it's time to adjust the balance of your closet so that it reflects your lifestyle.

In the sample charts below, the work clothes outweigh the social and leisure clothes, so any new purchases should be for these categories.

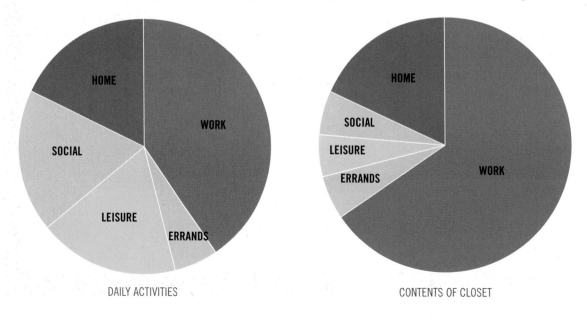

DAILY ACTIVITIES                    CONTENTS OF CLOSET

# CHECKLIST

Using the checklist below, note the color and style of the clothes that you already own. You can then determine what clothes you need to create your ideal closet. If you wish, make photocopies of the chart to use each time you overhaul your closet. You can also download a more detailed checklist from the **color me beautiful** website: www.colormebeautiful.co.uk
Enjoy taking inventory!

| | COLORS I HAVE | STYLES I HAVE | COLORS I NEED | STYLES I NEED |
|---|---|---|---|---|
| JACKETS | | | | |
| SKIRTS | | | | |
| PANTS | | | | |
| TOPS | | | | |
| DRESSES | | | | |
| COATS | | | | |
| UNDERWEAR | | | | |
| SHOES | | | | |
| HANDBAGS | | | | |
| SCARVES | | | | |
| BELTS | | | | |

# index

## A

accessories 181–3
  capsule closets 198–201
  City Chic style 161
  Classic style 157
  Creative style 151
  Dramatic style 153
  Natural style 159
  in pregnancy 185
  Romantic style 155
  wearing with black 107
all-over color 139
ankles 143
appropriate clothes 17
Arquette, Courtney Cox 82
average scale 138

## B

bags 182–3
  capsule closets 198–201
balanced body 113, 116
balanced waist 136
Beckham, Victoria 152
beige, psychology of 29
belts 182
black
  how to wear 106–8
  psychology of 29
black, alternatives to
  Clear and Cool 93
  Clear and Warm 89
  Cool and Clear 81
  Cool and Soft 77
  Deep and Cool 57
  Deep and Warm 53
  Light and Cool 45
  Light and Warm 41
  Soft and Cool 105
  Soft and Warm 101
  Warm and Clear 69
  Warm and Soft 65
Blanchett, Cate 34

blocks of color 139
blue, psychology of 30
blush 173, 174
body fat, genetics and 113
body shapes 16, 111–43
  proportions 136–7
  scale 138
  who can wear what 130–5
boots 183
bottoms, clothing details 142
bras 140, 180
brown, psychology of 29
Bruni-Sarkozy, Carla 160
business wear
  capsule closet 198–9
  Clear and Cool 92
  Clear and Warm 88
  Cool and Clear 80
  Cool and Soft 76
  Deep and Cool 56
  Deep and Warm 52
  Light and Cool 44
  Light and Warm 40
  Soft and Cool 104
  Soft and Warm 100
  Warm and Clear 68
  Warm and Soft 64
bustlines 140

## C

capsule closets 198–201
cardigans 200–1
casual wear
  capsule closet 200–1
  Clear and Cool 92
  Clear and Warm 88
  Cool and Clear 80
  Cool and Soft 76
  Deep and Cool 56
  Deep and Warm 52
  Light and Cool 44
  Light and Warm 40
  Soft and Cool 104
  Soft and Warm 100

  Warm and Clear 68
  Warm and Soft 64
chin shapes 165
chroma, color 25
City Chic style 146, 160–1, 189
clarity of color 25
Classic style 146, 156–7, 188
Clear 82–93
  Clear and Cool 90–3
  Clear and Warm 86–9
  color palette 84–5
  Cool and Clear 78–81
  investment buys 83
  Warm and Clear 66–9
  wearing black 109
Clinton, Hillary 156
closet, organizing 194–5
clothes
  capsule closets 198–201
  care of 197
  City Chic style 160–1
  Classic style 156–7
  Creative style 150–1
  details 140–3
  Dramatic style 152–3
  dresses 106, 135
  evening glamour 186–9
  flattering color combinations 139
  Full Hourglass shape 118–19
  Inverted Triangle shape 122–3
  jackets 131
  Lean Column shape 124–5
  Natural style 158–9
  Neat Hourglass shape 116–17
  organizing your closet 194–5
  pants 134
  planning for future 202–3
  in pregnancy 184–5
  Rectangle shape 126–7
  Romantic style 154–5
  Round shape 128–9
  shopping 196–7
  skirts 133
  tops 132

Triangle shape 120–1
underwear 180
vacation packing 190–1
coats, capsule closet 198–9
color 16
   City Chic style 161
   Classic style 157
   Clear color palette 84–5
   color analysis 26–7
   color confidence 32–3
   color theory 24–5
   coloring 22
   Cool color palette 72–3
   Creative style 151
   deep color palette 48–9
   Dramatic style 153
   flattering combinations 139
   Light color palette 36–7
   Natural style 159
   psychology of 28–31
   Romantic style 155
   Soft color palette 96–7
   Warm color palette 60–1
confidence 12–13, 32–3
Cool 25, 70–82
   Clear and Cool 90–3
   color palette 72–3
   Cool and Clear 78–81
   Cool and Soft 74–7
   Deep and Cool 54–7
   Inverted Triangle shape 123
   investment buys 71
   Light and Cool 42–5
   skin color 32
   Soft and Cool 102–5
   wearing black 109
cool-weather combinations
   Clear and Cool 92
   Clear and Warm 88
   Cool and Clear 80
   Cool and Soft 76
   Deep and Cool 56
   Deep and Warm 52
   Light and Cool 44

   Light and Warm 40
   Soft and Cool 104
   Soft and Warm 100
   Warm and Clear 68
   Warm and Soft 64
Creative style 146, 150–1, 186

**D**

Deep 46–57
   color palette 48–9
   Deep and Cool 54–7
   Deep and Warm 50–3
   investment buys 47
   wearing black 108
Dench, Judi 70
Deneuve, Catherine 146
depth of color 25
dominant coloring 32
Dramatic style 146, 152–3, 187
dresses 135
   capsule closets 198–200
   little black dress (LBD) 106
   in pregnancy 185
dry-cleaning 197
dyes, hair 25

**E**

earrings, and face shape 166–70
ears, shape 165
evening glamour 174, 186–9
eyebrows 173
eyeglasses, and face shape 165–70
eyelashes 173
eyes
   changes in coloring 27
   makeup 173, 174, 176
   shape 176

**F**

fabrics
   black 106, 107
   and color chroma 25
   Full Hourglass shape 119
   Inverted Triangle shape 123

   Lean Column shape 125
   Neat Hourglass shape 117
   Rectangle shape 127
   Round shape 129
   Triangle shape 121
face
   shape and proportion 164–70
   *see also* makeup
Fashion Academy of Los Angeles 24
fashion buys 196
footwear *see* boots; shoes
forehead, face shape 165
formal wear *see* business wear
foundation 172
Full Hourglass shape 114

**G**

genetics, body shapes 112–13
glamming up 174, 186–9
glasses, and face shape 165–70
grand scale 138
gray, psychology of 29
green, psychology of 31

**H**

hair
   changes in coloring 27
   City Chic style 161
   Classic style 157
   Clear and Cool 91
   Clear and Warm 87
   Cool and Clear 79
   Cool and Soft 75
   Creative style 151
   Deep and Cool 55
   Deep and Warm 51
   Dramatic style 153
   dyes 25
   evening glamour 189
   and face shape 165–70
   Light and Cool 43
   Light and Warm 39
   Natural style 159

Romantic style 155
Soft and Cool 103
Soft and Warm 99
Warm and Clear 67
Warm and Soft 63
hats 181
high-waisted shape 137
hourglass shape
    Full Hourglass shape 114, 118–19
    Neat Hourglass shape 113, 114,
       116–17
hue, color 25

**I**

Inverted Triangle
    body shape 115, 122–3
    face shape 169
investment buys 28, 147
    Clear 83
    Cool 71
    Deep 47
    Light 35
    shopping for 196
    Soft 95
    Warm 59
Itten, Johannes 24

**J**

jackets 131
    capsule closets 198–201
Jackson, Carole 24
jeans 200–1
jewelry 107, 181

**K**

Kidman, Nicole 146, 154

**L**

Lean Column shape 115, 124–5
legs
    clothing details 143
    proportions 136–7
Light 34–45
    color palette 36–7

investment buys 35
Light and Cool 42–5
Light and Warm 38–41
reflecting 25
wearing black 108
lips, shape 177
lipstick 173, 177
    evening makeup 174
    wearing with black 107
little black dress (LBD) 106
Lopez, Jennifer 112
low-waisted shape 137

**M**

MacArthur, Dame Ellen 146
makeup 171–9
    application techniques 172–3
    changing style 178–9
    City Chic style 161
    Classic style 157
    Clear and Cool 91
    Clear and Warm 87
    Cool and Clear 79
    Cool and Soft 75
    Creative style 151
    Deep and Cool 55
    Deep and Warm 51
    Dramatic style 153
    evening makeup 174, 189
    eyes 173, 174, 176
    and face shape 165–70
    Light and Cool 43
    Light and Warm 39
    lips 173, 174, 177
    Natural style 159
    Romantic style 155
    Soft and Cool 103
    Soft and Warm 99
    tools 171
    Warm and Clear 67
    Warm and Soft 63
    wearing with black 107
mascara 173
mixing colors

Clear and Cool 92–3
Clear and Warm 88–9
Cool and Clear 80–1
Cool and Soft 76–7
Deep and Cool 56–7
Deep and Warm 52–3
flattering combinations 139
Light and Cool 44–5
Light and Warm 40–1
Soft and Cool 104–5
Soft and Warm 100–1
Warm and Clear 68–9
Warm and Soft 64–5
Moore, Julianne 58
Munsell, Alfred 24–5

**N**

Natural style 146, 158–9, 188
Neat Hourglass shape 113, 114,
    116–17
necklines 141
nose shape 165

**O**

Obama, Michelle 46
organizing your closet 194–5
Osbourne, Sharon 146
oval face 166

**P**

panties 180
pants 134
    capsule closets 198–201
    in pregnancy 185
pantyhose 180
patterns
    Full Hourglass shape 119
    Lean Column shape 125
    Neat Hourglass shape 117
    Rectangle shape 127
    Round shape 129
    Triangle shape 121
personality *see* style personality
petite scale 138

pie charts, planning for future 202
pink, psychology of 30
Pooser, Doris 24
powder 172
pregnancy 184–5
profile, facial 164–5
proportion
    body shape 16, 136–7
    face shape 164–70
psychology of color 28–31
purple, psychology of 31

**R**

Rectangle
    body shape 115, 126–7
    face shape 168
red, psychology of 31
Rice, Condoleezza 146
Roberts, Julia 158
Romantic style 146, 154–5, 187
Round
    body shape 115, 128–9
    face shape 170

**S**

sandals 183
scale 16, 138
scarves 107, 182
secondary characteristics 32
shapes see body shapes
shoes 183
    details 143
    capsule closets 198–201
    care of 197
    in pregnancy 185
shopping 196–7
shoulder lines 141
skin
    changes in coloring 27
    skin adjusters 172
    skincare regimes 178–9
    see also makeup
skirts 133
    capsule closets 198–201

sleeve lengths 142
Soft 94–105
    color palette 96–7
    Cool and Soft 74–7
    investment buys 95
    Soft and Cool 102–5
    Soft and Warm 98–101
    Warm and Soft 62–5
    wearing black 109
special occasion wear
    Clear and Cool 92
    Clear and Warm 88
    Cool and Clear 80
    Cool and Soft 76
    Deep and Cool 56
    Deep and Warm 52
    Light and Cool 44
    Light and Warm 40
    Soft and Cool 104
    Soft and Warm 100
    Warm and Clear 68
    Warm and Soft 64
Spillane, Mary 24
square face 167
Stefani, Gwen 146
style personality 17, 145–61
suits, capsule closet 198–9

**T**

texture, wearing black 106
thighs, clothing details 143
tools, makeup 171
tops 132
    capsule closets 198–201
    in pregnancy 185
trends, following 17
Triangle
    body shape 114, 120–1
    Inverted Triangle face 169
    Inverted Triangle body shape
        115, 122–3
tummy, clothing details 143
two-color combinations see
    mixing colors

**U**

undertones, colors 25, 32
underwear 180, 189

**V**

vacation packing 190–1
value, color 25

**W**

waist, proportions 136–7
waistlines 142
Warm 58–69
    Clear and Warm 86–9
    color palette 60–1
    Deep and Warm 50–3
    investment buys 59
    Light and Warm 38–41
    skin colors 32
    Soft and Warm 98–101
    Warm and Clear 66–9
    Warm and Soft 62–5
    wearing black 108
warm colors 25
warm-weather combinations
    Clear and Cool 92
    Clear and Warm 88
    Cool and Clear 80
    Cool and Soft 76
    Deep and Cool 56
    Deep and Warm 52
    Light and Cool 44
    Light and Warm 40
    Soft and Cool 104
    Soft and Warm 100
    Warm and Clear 68
    Warm and Soft 64
well-dressed woman 16–17
Westwood, Vivienne 150
white, psychology of 30
Winslet, Kate 94

# acknowledgments

Little did we know when *Color Me Confident* was first published in 2006, that four years later we would be revisiting it and updating it. It is a real privilege to be able to go back and—hopefully—improve on what we have done before. Many thanks to the Hamlyn team, who extended the invitation to do so and who, as usual, have been most supportive within a very tight schedule—particularly Katy Denny who flies the **colour me beautiful** flag at all times.

Again, we asked willing **colour me beautiful** consultants to grace the pages of this book. They not only gave us their time but also brought in masses of clothes, and they are: Maureen Henderson, Sarah Kneafsey, Mandy Lehto, Ruth Murphy, Beth Price, and Louise Ravenscroft. Franca McBarron's picture from *Color Me Younger* also appears in this book. Friends very kindly joined in: Katy Denny, Ivy Harris, Fiona Wellins, and Ruth Wiseall could not be kept away. And just because we couldn't do without their original photographs, they are back in: Norma Couch, Ros Evans, Danni Meharg, and Angela Harris. Thank you to all those real, gorgeous women for their patience and enthusiasm in front of the camera.

We have worked with Jill Bay for many years and we are delighted that her illustrations are now in this edition.

All our thanks go to our support team of Audrey Hanna and Fiona Wellins. Audrey masterminded the shoot on our behalf at the risk of drowning in lists, while Fiona worked with the various public relations officers to make sure that the clothes arrived on time.

We are most grateful to all those people involved, to our colleagues at head office for their continued support, and to all the image consultants out there who use our books as their style bibles.

*Pat Henshaw and Veronique Henderson*

For more information on services, products, and how to become a consultant, contact **colour me beautiful**:

**UK and Headquarters for Europe, Africa and the Middle East**
66 The Business Centre,
15–17 Ingate Place,
London SW8 3NS
www.colourmebeautiful.co.uk
info@cmb.co.uk
t: +44 (0)20 7627 5211

**China**
www.qixincolor.com
**Finland**
www.colourmebeautiful.fi
**Ireland**
www.cmbireland.com
**Hong Kong**
www.colourmebeautiful.hk
**Netherlands, Germany & Belgium**
www.colourmebeautiful.nl
**Portugal**
www.cmb.com.pt
**Slovenia**
www.cmb.si
**South Africa**
www.colormebeautiful.co.za
**Spain**
www.colormebeautiful.es
**Sweden**
www.colormebeautiful.se
**USA**
www.colormebeautiful.com

## CLOTHES AND ACCESSORIES ACKNOWLEDGMENTS

**Betty Barclay** www.bettybarclay.co.uk
**Gil Bret** www.gilbret.co.uk
**LK Bennett** www.lkbennett.co.uk
**Spirit of the Andes**
www.spiritoftheandes.co.uk
**Vera Mont** www.veramont.co.uk

## PICTURE CREDITS

Special Photography: © **Octopus Publishing Group Limited**/Mike Prior

Other Photography:
**Alamy**/All Star Picture Library 27 right; /mediablitzimages (uk) Limited 185. **Corbis**/Rick Gomez 187 left; /Neil Guegan 186; /Charles Gullung 188 left; /Frank Trapper 26 top center, 58. **Getty Images**/DreamPictures 189; /Sean Gallup 26 bottom left, 46; /Ian Gavan 150; /Jeff Haynes/AFP 26 bottom center, 70; /Jon Kopaloff 26 top right, 82; /Peter Kramer 156; /Chris Polk/FilmMagic 26 top left, 32 bottom left, 34; /Stockbyte 190; /WireImage 158, 160, 184. **Masterfile** 187 right; /Jerzyworks 188 right. **Photoshot**/Omar Reyes/LANDOV 112 **Press Association Images**/Evan Agostini/AP 154. **Rex Features** 27 left; /Picture Perfect 26 bottom right, 94; /Nikos Vinieratos 152.

## FOR HAMLYN

**Executive Editor** Katy Denny
**Senior Editor** Charlotte Macey
**Deputy Creative Director** Karen Sawyer
**Designer** Mark Stevens
**Photographer** Mike Prior
**Hair and Make up** Stephen McIlmoyle
**Production Controller** Linda Parry